Defeating Diabetes

Brenda Davis, RD
Tom Barnard, MD

Healthy Living Publications
Summertown, Tennessee

Cover design: Warren Jefferson, Cynthia Holzapfel
Interior design: John Wincek
Editor: Karen Strauss

Published in the United States by
Healthy Living Publications

Printed in Canada

ISBN 1-57067-139-7

08   07   06   05   04   03   6   5   4   3

Davis, Brenda, 1959-
   Defeating diabetes / by Brenda Davis and Tom Barnard.
       p. cm.
Includes bibliographical references and index.
   ISBN 1-57067-139-7
   1. Diabetes–Popular works. 2. Diabetes–Diet therapy–Recipes. I. Barnard, Tom, 1948- II. Title.
   RC660.4.B37 2003
   616.4'62--dc21
                                        2002155993

Calculations for the nutritional analyses in this book are based on the average number of servings listed with the recipes and the average amount of an ingredient if a range is called for. Calculations are rounded up to the nearest gram. If two options for an ingredient are listed, the first one is used. Not included are fat used for frying (unless the amount is specified in the recipe), optional ingredients, or serving suggestions.

TABLE OF CONTENTS

Dedications

To my hero, my father, John Louis Charbonneau.

When I was a little girl, you were the smartest, bravest, and most generous person I knew—a real-live Santa Claus and superhero rolled into one. You were a remarkable repairman—fixing dolls, scooters, airplanes, and even broken hearts. You were a marvellous magician—transforming old bikes into fancy mustangs, back yards into skating rinks, and little girls into princesses. You were a tremendous teacher—imparting knowledge about algebra, biology, and the miracles of life and love.

Four decades have come and gone, and through each and every one, you have continued to amaze me more. I have grown to understand that you are no ordinary father, no ordinary man. Whatever part of me is a reflection of you, I treasure with all my heart and soul.

All my love,
Brenda

To my mother, Celia LaPardo Barnard.

Thank you for your grace and support throughout my life, which I feel even now, years after your passing.

To my sister, Dorothy Barnard Thompson

My "second" mother, my oldest living sister, Dorothy, thank you for all your help and support over the years. You are a great tower of strength for all of those in your family and your students who have numbered many over the years.

With love,
Tom

Acknowledgments

To our many teachers, professors, patients, and friends, our most humble gratitude. To everyone who gave of their time and energy to this project, we offer our heartfelt appreciation.

Sincere gratitude to those who made this book possible: Our editors Cynthia Holzapfel and Karen Strauss for invaluable contributions, dedication, and attention to detail; our publisher, Bob Holzapfel, and the many talented individuals at The Book Publishing Company: Gwynelle Dismukes, Warren and Barbara Jefferson, and Anna Pope. It is a pleasure and a privilege to work with each one of you, both professionally and personally.

Love and gratitude to family: Paul, Leena, and Cory Davis (Brenda's husband and children) for endless support, encouragement, and understanding. Sarah Elizabeth Shapiro Barnard (Tom's wife), carrying Ashoka (Tom and Sarah's son) at the time of this writing, for remarkable insights, connections to the Higher Self, and guidance of the Spirit. Sujata Star Barnard (Tom's daughter), for lessons about nutrition in the real world of a teenage girl, and for allowing me to steal some time away to write, even though we always had important things to discuss.

Deepest appreciation to our esteemed reviewers and advisors: David Jenkins, MD, Ph, DSc, for his kind support and tremendous ongoing work in the field of nutrition and health. Bruce Holub, PhD, for remarkable work in the field of fatty acid metabolism, and for insight and understanding regarding the effects of trans fatty acids. Dina Aronson, MS, RD, LDN, for detailed and most insightful reviews of chapters 2 and 5. Stephen Walsh, PhD for thought-provoking comments and suggestions for chapters 1, 2, and 10. Dennis Gorden, MEd, RD, and Sandra Hood, RD, for careful review of chapter 2. Patti Geil, MS, RD, FADA, CDE, for taking the time to carefully read through and comment on the manuscript. Ketti Goudey, MS, RD, for her thoughtful review of chapter 4. Allison Geiger, MA, for her detailed review of English and grammar. David Marcus for his insightful review of the entire book. Vesanto Melina, MS, RD, for ongoing advice and support.

Special thanks to our dear friends who contributed time, energy, valuable insights, and support: Margie Colclough, Butch and Laurie Johnston, Anthony Marr, Paul and Victoria Harrison.

Foreword

Tom Barnard and Brenda Davis have addressed the current epidemic of diabetes and related disorders with a lifestyle book that encourages a healthy body weight, exercise, and a good diet. Why is this important? It is estimated that by the year 2020, the diabetic population in Western nations will double. At this same time, there will be a proportionate increase in people who suffer the prediabetic state of insulin resistance and overweight, with many of the same risks, including cardiovascular disease and certain cancers, as shared by people with diabetes.

There is now an urgent need for strategies for change, since it is already estimated that 40% of those who enter middle age are overweight and at increased risk of diabetes. This book therefore aims at prevention of complications. What is new about the advice to follow a healthy diet? Tom and Brenda have taken up the challenge proved by current international and national agencies to eat a more plant-based diet, to eat more fruit and vegetables, and eat fewer calories in total. Accordingly, their diets are balanced—rich in the vitamins, minerals, and phytochemicals which protect from chronic disease—are calorie-reduced, and, at the same time, palatable. Added to this, they have tried to make them environmentally friendly and sustainable, and one can clearly see the comprehensiveness of their dietary advice.

Their approach to diet and diabetes is, therefore, new and contains what the diabetic and nondiabetic need to know to stay healthy. Therefore, it is very much a book for the 21st century and worth the investment. Congratulations to them for putting such a book together.

Professor David Jenkins, MD
University of Toronto

CHAPTER 1

Can You Defeat Diabetes?

*T*om: *Standing in the hospital room at the St. Francis Medical Center outside New York City, I remember vividly the concern I felt for my sister. As a doctor for several decades, I was used to the chaos of hospitals and the close atmosphere of the hospital waiting room, with the members of different families and cultures mixing in a cramped, anxiety-filled space. My sister awaited heart bypass surgery there, her worried son with her. Standing in a hospital gown, leaning on her IV pole for support, she looked older, battle-worn; chest pain would frequently interrupt our brief walks down brightly lit hospital corridors.*

Waiting there, watching my sister's pain and fear and my nephew's desperate wish to ease his mother's suffering, I wondered to myself, could we have reversed her chest pain and minimized her

1

risk of heart attack by getting her to eat a better diet and take better care of herself? I would have stood in front of a moving truck if it would have helped my sister at that moment, but in fact, I did something practical. I made arrangements to have good food brought to her and to have her work with Dr. Dean Ornish's Reversal of Heart Disease program once she had come through bypass surgery. Although my sister was in the hospital waiting for critical heart bypass surgery, the disease that was trying to kill her had been quietly and efficiently at work for years, with few outward signs. You see, it wasn't hereditary or congenital heart disease that was killing my sister—it was diabetes.

The diabetes that my sister had developed, type 2 (also called adult-onset), had shown no obvious symptoms, no sudden, dangerously high blood sugars or diabetic comas. It had insidiously crept up on her over the years, damaging her arterial walls and her nerves, leaving my once-vibrant sibling impaired, injured, and in fear for her life whenever crippling chest pain would seize her. Following her surgery, my sister embarked on a renewed commitment to living, following the type of diet we recommend in this book, and enhancing her quality of life and her enjoyment of living in the process. I am deeply grateful that my sister is still with us, years after this crisis threatened to end her life. She went from a prognosis of death from diabetic complications to a plan for living well and prospering.

I was determined to write this book with my friend Brenda Davis, knowing that, without an aggressive plan for stopping the disease in its tracks, my sister, and millions of others with type 2 diabetes, would have their lives cut short from the complications of the disease. This book is that plan.

WHAT IS DIABETES?

Although diabetes has been known since ancient times, it is only in the last twenty years that the disease has become a worldwide epidemic, not only in adults, but also in children. Sadly, one type of diabetes, type 2, has become a disease of nutritional extravagance. As we eat more calories and exercise less, the disease damages and then destroys our bodies from the inside out, in an insidious, long-term process that can be likened to drops of water quietly and systematically wearing away a stone.

The term diabetes dates back to ancient times when healers, attempting to diagnose a person who was wasting away, would taste their urine for sweetness. The word derives from the Greek for "siphon," an apt description of the excessive urination that is a common symptom of diabetes. Several centuries later the name was expanded to diabetes mellitus, mellitus being the Latin word for "honey" or "sweet tasting." In people with diabetes, excess blood sugar, or glucose, spills into the urine, hence the sweetness noticed by the ancient healers.

Although diabetes was an uncommon diagnosis in ancient times, it meant a death sentence for its victims. Treatment options were numerous and varied, including botanical remedies and starvation diets. Some healers managed to prolong life in their patients by a few weeks or perhaps even months, but nothing offered any real hope for survival, nothing, that is, until the role insulin plays in the body was discovered by researchers at the University of Toronto. Collected from the pancreases of slaughtered cows, insulin was first used clinically in 1921, significantly prolonging the life of a young boy with type 1 diabetes.

Defining Diabetes

Diabetes is a disease in which the body fails to produce or properly use insulin. Insulin is a protein hormone secreted by the islets of Langerhans in the pancreas. It helps the body use carbohydrates, which are the starches and sugars found in the food we eat. The oldest known form of diabetes, type 1, is characterized by the destruction of the insulin-producing cells of the pancreas, so that the body no longer secretes insulin, or produces negligible amounts. Type 1 has also been called juvenile-onset diabetes, because its victims are most often children and juveniles. It has also been called insulin-dependent diabetes because people who have it rely on daily insulin, administered via injection or a pump, for survival.

Type 1 is an autoimmune disorder caused when the body mistakenly produces antibodies that attack and damage the pancreas. It is not known what triggers antibody production, although viruses and other environmental factors are suspected. Other risk factors include genetic predisposition. The onset of type 1 is usually sudden. Currently only 5 to 10 percent of people with diabetes suffer from type 1.

Untreated, a person with type 1 diabetes will develop hyperglycemia, or high blood sugar, characterized by increasing fatigue, then confusion, and eventually coma. Even with insulin treatment, people with type 1 must take care to avoid a host of related health problems ranging from blindness, premature heart attack and stroke, kidney failure, nerve damage, and poor wound healing, which can result in amputation of the toes, feet, or lower legs.

The vast majority of people with diabetes throughout the world suffer from type 2 diabetes. Unfortunately, type 2 has become a worldwide epidemic, not only in adults but also in young people, particularly in affluent countries. In the year 2000, a four-year-old child in Arkansas was diagnosed with type 2 diabetes, and it is not uncommon these days to hear of ten-year-old children being diagnosed. Although type 1, or juvenile diabetes, is still the most common form of diabetes in children, type 2 is rapidly gaining ground.

Type 2 diabetes occurs either when the body is unable to make enough insulin to process the amount of glucose (blood sugar) in the blood or when it cannot effectively use the amount of insulin being produced. Type 2 used to be called adult-onset diabetes or noninsulin-dependent diabetes because, until recently, it occurred most often in aging, overweight adults. It accounts for 90 to 95 percent of all diabetes cases today. The onset is gradual and usually begins as a series of symptoms that are often overlooked or misdiagnosed. In addition, for reasons that are still unclear to us, the body may not utilize the insulin it makes, a condition that may develop for years prior to the actual onset of elevations of blood glucose. This condition causes significant changes to body chemistry that contribute to the slow, but steady, development of high blood pressure and heart disease, even years before any diagnosis of diabetes is made.

Type 2 diabetes is associated with being overweight, with having high blood sugar associated with poor eating habits and lack of exercise, and also with high cholesterol, high triglycerides (blood fats), and high blood pressure. It is a disease of excess (too many calories), and lifestyle (not enough exercise). Untreated, type 2 diabetes leads to debilitating health problems similar to type 1 diabetes.

A much less common form of diabetes, gestational diabetes, is a temporary condition that occurs during pregnancy, ending with delivery of the baby. It occurs during 2 to 4 percent of all pregnancies. Although gestational diabetes ends after delivery, 50 percent of the women who had gestational diabetes will develop type 2 diabetes later in life. Their children also are at greater risk for type 2. Untreated, gestational diabetes can harm the fetus's heart and liver, and can result in serious birth defects or stillbirth if the mother's blood sugar is not controlled.

Type 2 diabetes is often insidious. In fact, about half of those with type 2 diabetes don't know they have it because so many of the individual symptoms could be indicative of other problems. If you or someone you care about is experiencing several of the following symptoms, testing for diabetes is very important.

Classic Symptoms of Diabetes

- Frequent urination
- Excessive thirst
- Extreme hunger
- Unusual weight loss

- Extreme fatigue
- Irritability
- Blurred vision
- Poor wound healing

If you suspect diabetes, your doctor will order one or more blood tests to confirm the diagnosis. You may want to test your blood sugar with a home glucose monitor and then follow up with your health care provider. If your tests are positive, they can be repeated on a different day to confirm the diagnosis, although if the first tests are very high, there is usually little doubt that they are accurate.

THE EVOLUTION OF AN EPIDEMIC

Type 2 diabetes can quietly wreak havoc inside a person's body long before symptoms become serious. In recent years, experts have come to realize that people go through months and even years of various prediabetic conditions before being diagnosed with type 2 diabetes. Prediabetes is now recognized as a medical condition of higher than normal blood sugar affecting more than sixteen million Americans. Without treatment, people with prediabetes are headed down a rocky road to full-blown type 2 diabetes.

For many people, the first step to diabetes is insulin resistance, in some cases even before diabetes can be diagnosed. Insulin resistance can also be part of a syndrome leading to prediabetes and full-blown type 2. Insulin resistance syndrome is characterized by high blood pressure, abdominal fat, high blood fats, low HDL or "good" cholesterol, obesity, and high uric acid associated with increased heart attacks. Insulin resistance syndrome is also sometimes called metabolic syndrome or syndrome X. Insulin resistance increases your chances of having a heart attack. It can be corrected with weight loss and exercise.

Markers of Metabolic Syndrome

According to the National Institutes of Health (NIH), metabolic syndrome is present if any three or more symptoms are present:

- a waist measurement of at least 40 inches for men and 35 inches for women
- triglyceride levels of at least 150 mg/dL (1.7 mmol/L)
- HDL levels of less than 40 mg/dL (1 mmol/L) in men and less than 50 mg/dL (1.3 mmol/L) in women
- blood pressure of at least 135/80
- blood sugar of at least 110 mg/dL (6.1 mmol/L) in the fasting state

To understand how insulin resistance works, imagine that cells in our bodies have "gate-keepers" called insulin receptors. Insulin, the key hormone that allows glucose to enter the cells, is produced by the beta cells of the pancreas. Insulin's job is to travel from the pancreas to cells all over the body, unlocking the cells so glucose can enter. After glucose enters, the cells can immediately use it for energy, store it for rapid use later on, or convert it to fat for use as energy even later.

When the gate-keeper cells function normally, they are sensitive to insulin and respond, taking up glucose or blood sugar from the blood. If the gate-keepers are insensitive to insulin, they do not "open up," and glucose or sugar remains in the blood stream, despite insulin being present. The glucose is not burned off for fuel, and its continued presence stimulates production of more insulin. Because the body is not using insulin properly, the pancreas is "confused" and keeps pumping more out in an effort to compensate. The body remains stubbornly insensitive to increasing amounts of insulin, eventually becoming resistant. As a result of resistance to insulin, blood sugar is not burned or metabolized, and blood sugar rises, leading to diabetes and a host of other health problems, including heart disease.

A primary factor in insulin resistance is being overweight. Obesity plus insulin resistance equals "diabesity," the new face of the current epidemic of type 2 diabetes. When a person's weight is in healthy ranges, fat cells control insulin by releasing hormones that curb the appetite when blood glucose levels are high. When the person responds to these natural appetite suppressants and eats only the amount needed to fuel the body, there is little excess blood sugar that needs to be stored as fat.

When a person overeats and overrides the body's hormonal appetite suppressants day after day, the cells are continuously bathed in large amounts of insulin. This causes them to resist absorbing glucose and processing it to provide the body with energy. Instead, high insulin levels cause the cells to multiply in order to store the extra glucose, and we end up with extra fat cells. Because muscle tissue is a more efficient fuel burner than fat tissue, the more muscle tissue we have, the more fuel the body can burn, and the less likely that excess, unburned calories will accumulate as fat. However, the more fat tissue we have, the more likely it is that we will develop the vicious cycle of insulin resistance that increases high blood sugar, as well as encourages storage of excess fat.

As you can see, weight control is a vitally important weapon when it comes to controlling diabetes, as is exercise. But there are other factors that must be considered as well.

What Does Insulin Resistance and the Road to Diabetes Feel Like?

A second important weapon in fighting diabetes is to recognize the warning signals of insulin resistance and metabolic syndrome before damage occurs or before we become overtly diabetic. For the most part, insulin resistance feels and looks tired. It feels like our memory doesn't work, that we "run out of gas" in the middle of things, both physically and mentally. If our cells don't respond to insulin normally, they don't get their proper supply of fuel in a timely manner. And if more and more insulin is required to process a meal, higher insulin levels will engender sluggishness, much like the feeling of eating a very big meal. That sluggishness, that overwhelming fatigue, becomes more and more common as insulin resistance and, ultimately, diabetes develops.

Along with the symptoms of insulin resistance and high blood sugar, we should be aware of the symptoms of low blood sugar, or hypoglycemia. We've all heard of or even experienced the occasional episode of low blood sugar, perhaps after skipping a meal or waiting too long between meals. As mentioned above, after undergoing an exaggerated insulin response to glucose metabolized from our foods, we might also experience sluggishness right after a meal, caused by rising glucose and insulin levels. With this exaggerated insulin response there may follow a rapid movement of glucose into cells, leading to a drop in blood sugar and the development of low blood sugar or reactive hypoglycemia. This blood sugar drop compounds sluggishness and adds another reaction to an already volatile mix as the body attempts to keep blood sugar levels from falling too low. A hormonal response by the body will restore blood sugar, but at the same time cause symptoms of adrenal hormone excess: anxiety and tremulousness, irritability, sweating, and dilation of the pupils. As you can see, one reaction leads to another reaction, all of which adds stress and strain to the body. Eventually, the toll taken on the body trying to regulate its insulin response to out-of-control blood sugars results in diabetes and all of its varied and debilitating complications.

The Slippery Slope of Diabetic Complications

We are all going to age, we will tire once in awhile, and we all have to die of something. However, diabetes is being diagnosed in people at a younger and younger age. Hand in hand with insulin resistance and the rise in blood sugars comes a dangerous physiological price tag, and the earlier in life diabetes occurs, the longer our bodies will have to pay this price. Not only are our bodies exposed to high insulin levels and the resulting weight gain, but there appears to be an increased risk for damage to important molecules that control other body functions. Pain and inflammation increase, and damage to tissues accelerates. Even a small elevation in blood sugars results in the body's cells being bathed in sugary molecules.

These sugar molecules are actually sticky, causing our tissues to "caramelize," as it were, with sugars sticking to proteins and enzymes, bridging spaces between connective tissue layers. Our arteries stiffen, the lenses of our eyes become less flexible, and we are exposed to the effects of living in a sugary, syrupy body fluid. This change in the environment in which our cells operate has profound implications. We are more likely to develop atherosclerosis, hardening of the arteries, throughout our bodies, leading to a significant increase in the risk of heart disease, stroke, and kidney disease. Sugar molecules also attach themselves to the nerves in our legs, deadening our ability to feel and sense heat and pain properly. It's as if a type of internal rusting is corroding the wiring leading to the central switchboard of our brain and nervous system. Even the wires controlling heart rhythm are not spared, increasing the chance for arrhythmias from restriction of blood supply to the heart muscle, and from the damage that occurs to the pacemaker cells of the heart and the conduction wiring in the heart bundles and muscles themselves.

Finally, our ability to fight infection dwindles. With elevated sugar levels, immune cells go from being vigilant defenders to being sluggish, depressed, and simply "stunned" in the face of invading germs, viruses, and fungi. That is why yeast infections are so common with elevated blood sugars. Not only does sweetened body fluid and tissue offer an ideal environment for yeast and fungal growth, but immune surveillance mechanisms simply do not work well in the face of rising insulin and sugar levels.

Type 2 Diabetes...FAST FACTS

- Number of North Americans with diabetes: more than 18 million

- Number of new cases diagnosed annually in North America: nearly 1 million

- Increase in incidence of diabetes in North America between 1958 and 1997: sixfold

- Increase in type 2 diabetes among people in their 30s between 1990 and 1998: 70%

- Percent of North American adults with diabetes: about 8%

- North Americans with insulin resistance: about 25%

- Increase in number of obese children compared to 1975: triple

- North Americans above 65 years of age with diabetes: about 18%

- Risk of cardiovascular disease in people with diabetes vs. those without diabetes: 2 to 4 times higher

- Risk of stroke in people with diabetes vs. those without diabetes: 2 to 4 times higher

- People with diabetes who also have high blood pressure: 60 to 65%

- People with diabetes who also have mild to severe diabetic nerve damage: 60 to 70%

- Risk of diabetes in people of aboriginal descent compared with the general population: 3 to 5 times higher

- Children and teens with newly diagnosed diabetes who are type 2: 33%

We can detect these problems early if we look hard enough. If we find ourselves fatigued and urinating frequently, a random blood sugar test should be given. If the test is not definitive and there is still some concern, a test of glucose metabolism is warranted, using either a measured amount of glucose (called a glucose load) or simply checking the blood glucose level after a meal. However this might not tell the whole story, as insulin levels might be high well before any discernible rise in blood glucose after eating. A glucose tolerance test that measures insulin levels both before and after taking a glucose sample could be an even better diagnostic tool to prevent future damage.

We are just beginning to appreciate the importance of a rise in triglycerides after eating as another risk factor for arterial disease. Not only is a rise in blood sugar damaging to tissues in the body, but so is an elevation of triglycerides, especially when there is glucose intolerance or insulin resistance. High glucose levels inhibit the enzymes that break down triglycerides so that these fats accumulate in the blood and promote atherosclerosis.

All of these changes in metabolism indicate the body's growing inability to process carbohydrates efficiently and are therefore associated with an increase in cardiovascular disease. With insulin becoming less effective in the body, not only will we begin to see the effects of rising sugar levels, but blood fats like triglycerides and cholesterol will begin to accumulate, especially after a meal. This will lead to more time when body tissues are awash in a sugary, fat-enriched serum.

Metabolic Obesity

Because the symptoms of diabetes might at first indicate other health problems, the disease is not always easy to diagnose and is often missed or overlooked in its early stages. To confuse matters even more, it is possible for a person to be thin, with relatively little body fat, and still be insulin resistant. This condition is known as being metabolically obese. The culprit could be abnormal molecules that modern science has introduced into our food to enhance its flavors and resistance to spoilage. Our bodies must try to cope with these foreign substances, which some researchers now believe are a trigger of insulin resistance.

One of the main reasons food spoils or goes rancid is the oxidation or breakdown of the fats in it. Modern food science tried to "improve" our food supply by making it safer from spoilage, but instead created other unanticipated health problems. One of these is metabolic obesity—or what could be called hydrogenation havoc. Chemically altered fats, called hydrogenated fats, take an inherently healthful food such as unsaturated vegetable oil and combine it with hydrogen, hardening or solidifying the oil to make it shelf-stable. During hydrogenation, other fats, called trans fats or trans fatty acids, also are created. These altered fats do not break down easily and resist spoilage, helping make foods taste and appear fresh even after weeks on the grocery shelves.

Hydrogenated and trans fats are found in vegetable shortening and margarine, as well as hundreds of food products ranging from baked goods to frozen entrées. They also might be responsible for decreasing our body's inherent ability to react to our insulin hormones properly. In the Nurses' Health Study, done to follow the development of chronic disease in 80,000 nurses over 15 years, hydrogenated fats were strongly associated with the risk of developing diabetes as an adult. While less spoilage in our foods may sound like a desirable, even innocent goal, the reality is that these abnormal fats are probably unsuited for the basic vital operations of our cellular machinery.

It is possible that hydrogenated fat molecules "dumb down" our cells, changing the structure and shape of the cell membranes so that even a small molecule like insulin finds itself unable to use the key that fits the lock of the gatekeeper cells. Unable to unlock the cells, glucose remains in the blood instead of being burned for fuel. Hampering this wonderful gatekeeper and key system, which is vitally responsible for our metabolic efficiency, and indeed our very survival, is dangerous. So, eliminating hydrogenated and partially hydrogenated fats from the diet so that our cells can accept and process insulin normally is part of a good strategy for avoiding insulin resistance and diabetes itself.

RISK ASSESSED, RISK AVERTED

Now that we have a better understanding of the different types of diabetes and the causes of type 2 diabetes, it becomes easier to accurately predict and analyze risk. If we can do a better job understanding who is most at risk, we can do more to preempt that risk!

Because we are experiencing type 2 diabetes in epidemic proportions now, we are focusing most of our strategies in this book on dealing with this form of the disease. But these strategies will also improve the quality of life for people with type 1 diabetes, and will reduce the risks for mothers with gestational diabetes and their unborn children.

As the *New England Journal of Medicine* reported in 2002, the treatments for insulin resistance, prediabesity, and diabetes emphasize the broad benefits of the following treatment tools:

- diet and exercise,
- stress management,
- and a more proactively healthful outlook on life.

These are the tools we'll teach you to employ in your journey to defeating diabetes. Not only are these interventions effective in preventing and treating diabetes and the trend to diabetes, but studies have confirmed that they can be as effective as diabetes medications—with broader benefits and fewer side effects. Certainly, diet and exercise should be the foundation of a coordinated approach to healing from diabetes. We also believe that good spiritual health can lead to better physical health, so in addition to information on the physical care of diabetes, we'll give you some practical tips for your soul.

The goals of this book are to help you achieve normal levels of blood sugars and blood fats both before and after meals. We also want to help you aim for normal blood pressure readings—a systolic pressure of 120 and a diastolic pressure of 80—eliminating any deleterious effect on your heart, kidneys, and arterial walls, as well as your central nervous system. The best way to achieve this is with the comprehensive lifestyle and life-altering approaches you'll find in the next several chapters.

There may be times when medications are helpful or necessary, despite our best efforts to live a diabetes-defeating lifestyle. For people whose type 2 diabetes has already progressed to dangerous levels, medications can help bring their disease under control quickly to prevent further tissue damage. Newer and safer medicines for reducing and normalizing blood sugar and blood fat elevations are being introduced all the time. In particular, losartan and irbesartan appear to offer some protection from metabolic syndrome. Once their condition is under control, the broader benefits of diet and exercise can help people defeat their diabetes. They can take what is useful from a basic lifestyle approach in combination with the best and newest medicines that research has to offer to achieve the best chance for success.

The good news is that insulin resistance, prediabetes, and type 2 diabetes itself are highly treatable, and often even reversible. And given that the problem of "diabesity" is growing among our children, as well as within our adult population, we need to know how to recognize the problem as it is developing and how to change our lives for the better.

~ ~ ~ ~ ~ ~ ~ ~ ~ ~ ~

Tom: Recently, a young patient reminded me of just how imperative it is to make healthful lifestyle choices from a very early age. Brendan was brought in by his mother, who was worried that this overweight champion video game player was far too tired for fourteen years of age. He did seem abnormally fatigued and lacking in motivation, and I wondered if it was a "teen thing" or whether he might be experimenting with drugs or perhaps dealing with depression. When we had a chance to talk, he commented that his sleep was interrupted at night by having to urinate frequently. In school, he added, he often needed to leave class to visit the restroom. At 5'11" and 230 pounds, Brendan was a big youngster, and much of his bulk was centered around his abdomen, a spare tire of fat.

With these clues, I now had a pretty good idea what ailed Brendan. When we had the chance to check his blood sugar in my office, my hunch was confirmed. At age fourteen, Brendan was diabetic—not the usual childhood diabetic with hugely elevated sugars, but what we had always called adult-onset diabetes, or type 2. He was able to make lots of insulin in his pancreas; it was just that he was overweight and not active enough. His body couldn't efficiently utilize all of the insulin it was producing to metabolize the blood sugar from all the food he ate. His fat tissue reacted to this insulin like a sponge by enlarging and storing more fat, while the muscle cells in his body were so overwhelmed by insulin, they could only sluggishly respond to the blood sugar that flooded his system. When his body drastically increased the amount of insulin it produced to overcome the insensitivity the muscle cells displayed, the result was a disaster. Because insulin is a storage hormone and drives the body to store calories as fat if enough fuel isn't being burned through vigorous physical activity, more and more fat was created from the fuel that Brendan would take in with his meals.

Really, the biggest hurdle for Brendan was to recognize that this was the beginning of a long, downhill slide, but that the solution was simple enough. Like Mark Twain said, "If you don't change directions, you will wind up where you are heading." And fortunately, Brendan was alert, interested, and motivated to take control over the circumstances that were leading him into this difficult situation. I worked with him to develop an understanding of blood sugar and insulin balance issues and what causes resistance to the effects of insulin in our bodies. Not only did he get it, he picked up the ball from me and ran toward the goal of better health.

Happily, when I saw Brendan a few weeks later, he was already losing weight, had joined the local gym, and had decided that playing soccer on the school team was better than Final Fantasy and other video games, at least for part of his day. He was moving toward a better lifestyle, one that would provide for good health for years to come. And his game plan—Eat Well, Live Well, Be Calm, Be Kind—is described in the chapters that follow.

CHAPTER 2

Diabetes & the Diet Connection

T he words diabetes and diet fit together like a ball and glove. It's commonly believed that people with diabetes are condemned to a lifelong diabetic diet. Most imagine a very rigid regime with complicated exchange lists, countless prohibited foods, special diet products, and tools for weighing and measuring everything. While people dread diabetes and the prospect of daily insulin injections, many dread the thought of having to follow a diabetic diet even more.

It may come as quite a surprise to learn that people with type 2 diabetes can manage their diet without exchange lists or food scales. We now have sufficient evidence to support the case for a far easier and remarkably more effective way of tackling this disease.

HEALTHY LIFESTYLES...OUR MOST POWERFUL ALLY

There is one thing that we know with absolute certainty: the difference in rates of type 2 diabetes among various populations is huge. Some populations living traditional lifestyles, with high levels of physical activity and plant-based diets (e.g., the Bantu in Tanzania and the Mapuche in Chile), have rates of type 2 diabetes that are close to zero. On the other hand, traditional peoples who now live more like typical North Americans with sedentary lifestyles and affluent, meat-centered, processed-food diets, have rates of type 2 diabetes that are upwards of 50 percent (e.g., the Pima Indians of Arizona and the Micronesians of Nauru). These high-risk populations have amazingly efficient metabolisms, finely tuned for survival—in other words, their genes are programmed to withstand famine, and when faced with a constant supply of calories, this efficiency works against them, causing obesity and diabetes. The million-dollar question becomes: If affected individuals renounce their affluent diet and sedentary lifestyle in favor of a traditional high-fiber, plant-based diet and a vigorous exercise regime, will the disease resolve itself?

Over two decades ago a rather unique study was designed to answer this very question. In this study, ten middle-aged aborigines from Western Australia with type 2 diabetes and obesity were returned to their traditional hunter-gatherer lifestyle in northwestern Australia for seven weeks. Physical activity shot up, and fat intake plummeted from about 40 to 13 percent of calories. The study participants lost an average of almost eighteen pounds. Fasting blood sugar dropped 43 percent. Since this work, other researchers have produced similar impressive results. One study placed twenty obese native Hawaiians on a traditional low-fat, high-unrefined-carbohydrate diet for three weeks. Fasting blood sugar levels dropped almost 25 percent; weight dropped an average of seventeen pounds, and cholesterol, triglycerides, and blood pressure all fell significantly.

Similar interventions in the general population have provided equally impressive results. In one study, thirteen men with type 2 diabetes were put on a high-carbohydrate, high-fiber diet for two weeks. All five men on diabetes medications, and four men on insulin were able to discontinue their use. Fasting blood sugars dropped, as did cholesterol and triglyceride levels. A larger study of more than 650 people with type 2 diabetes showed similar results, with 71 percent of the participants on oral medications and 39 percent of those on insulin able to stop. Participants also enjoyed improved fasting blood sugars, blood pressure, and cholesterol levels, as well as weight loss. Still another 12-week study compared those on a conventional American Diabetic Association (ADA) diet with those on a very low-fat, vegan (meat, egg, and dairy free), whole foods diet. The vegan group reduced its fasting blood sugar levels by 28 percent, almost 60 percent more than the ADA group. They also had almost twice the reduction in body weight and HbA1c (a measurement of how much glucose has attached to protein in our red blood cells—see the A1c test on page 180). Two-thirds of those in the vegan group were able to lower the amount of diabetes medication, while medication remained unchanged in the ADA group.

The success of these trials is hard to ignore, especially considering the high carbohydrate content of these diets (all over 70 percent of calories), as compared to conventional ADA diets with about 45 to 50 percent of calories from carbohydrates. Most people would expect such carbohydrate-loaded programs to wreak havoc with blood sugars. What spared the participants of these studies? There is no doubt it was the package the carbohydrates came in—whole plant foods, loaded with fiber.

> For many years, high intakes of carbohydrates have been thought of as unsafe for people with diabetes. The critical point that is often overlooked when considering the effects of carbohydrates on blood sugar is that the source of carbohydrate may be as important a consideration as the amount of carbohydrate consumed. When high-carbohydrate diets are shown to adversely affect blood sugar control and triglyceride levels, the sources of those carbohydrates are predictable: low-fiber, refined foods such as white bread, processed cereals, white rice, white pasta, pretzels, and baked goods. When high-carbohydrate diets are shown to favorably impact blood sugar control and triglycerides, the carbohydrate sources are equally predictable: high-fiber, whole, unprocessed plant foods such as whole grains, legumes, vegetables, fruits, nuts, and seeds.

It makes us wonder if current conventional diets for people with type 2 diabetes (less than 30 percent of calories from fat, less than 10 percent from saturated fat, and 20 to 35 grams of fiber per day) provide our best possible defense. While we know that these programs are moderately effective at controlling diabetes, more aggressive approaches appear to offer significantly greater benefits. High-fiber, plant-based diets are clearly the direction to head, although questions remain about the best makeup of these diets:

- How much fat should people with diabetes consume?

- What types of fat are the most healthful?

- What kinds of carbohydrates are best?

- How much fiber is needed to provide maximum benefit for glycemic control?

- What type of diet best supports weight loss?

These questions are best answered by examining the primary goals of diet therapy for people with type 2 diabetes.

> While current conventional diabetic diets are moderately effective, simple, unprocessed plant-based diets appear significantly more effective in both the prevention and treatment of diabetes.

GOALS OF DIET THERAPY

The ultimate goal in treating type 2 diabetes is to restore insulin function by overcoming insulin resistance. This is accomplished by major diet and lifestyle changes—primarily, increased physical activity and weight loss. There are three primary goals of diet therapy:

1. To protect against heart disease;

2. To promote healthy body weights;

3. To achieve and maintain good blood sugar control.

The purpose of these goals is to reduce both long- and short-term complications of diabetes. This includes diseases of the eye, kidney, nerves, heart, and blood vessels and the improvement of quality of life and overall health. We will examine the evidence and determine what type of diet best accomplishes each of these goals.

Goal #1: Heart Disease Protection

What diet best supports heart health? The diet most commonly recommended for the prevention and treatment of heart disease is the American Heart Association (AHA) "heart healthy" or "prudent" diet (less than 30 percent of calories from fat, 10 percent from saturated fat, and 300 mg cholesterol). While this diet goes a long way toward reducing the risk of heart disease, its effectiveness as a treatment for heart disease has been less than impressive, with cholesterol reductions averaging a modest 5 to 6 percent. More profound results have come from two seemingly opposite eating patterns: very low-fat vegetarian diets, and relatively high-fat Mediterranean diets.

Very Low-Fat Vegetarian Diets

Very low-fat vegetarian and vegan diets have been shown to be powerful allies in preventing and treating heart disease. Several researchers have demonstrated that not only do these diets surpass the usual cholesterol reduction seen in AHA diets, they can often reverse the course of the disease.

The most well recognized of these studies is the groundbreaking Lifestyle Heart Trial conducted by Dr. Dean Ornish. In this study, people with serious heart disease were put on a program including a very low-fat vegetarian diet, stress management, aerobic exercise, and group therapy. Ornish's group was compared with a control group following an AHA diet and exercise program. After one year, Ornish's experimental group had a drop of almost 38 percent in LDL cholesterol compared to only 6 percent in the control group. Angina (chest pain) fell by 91 percent in the experimental group, while it increased by 165 percent in the control group. An impressive 82 percent of the experimental group experienced some reversal of their disease, while in the control group the disease continued to progress.

In another study conducted by Dr. Caldwell Esselstyn of the Cleveland Clinic, eleven patients followed a very low-fat vegetarian diet, with cholesterol-lowering medication. Seventy percent of the participants experienced a reversal of their disease. In the eight years prior to the study, these patients experienced a total of forty-eight cardiac events (such as heart attacks), while during the twelve years of the study only one person had an event.

The results of these and other studies have made very low-fat, plant-based diets extremely attractive to those seeking to prevent or treat coronary artery disease.

High-Fat, Mediterranean-Style Diets

Many people assume that while high-fat diets might be effective in controlling blood sugar (because they are lower in carbohydrates), these diets would be damaging to heart health. This is not necessarily the case. Studies suggest that some types of higher-fat diets can actually protect the heart. The most significant of these is the Lyon Heart Study with 605 participants (all of whom had previously suffered a heart attack). Participants were assigned to follow either an AHA heart-healthy diet (303 patients) or a Mediterranean-style diet (302 patients). While the differences in total fat were very small, the Mediterranean

What does a Mediterranean diet look like?

Plentiful vegetables, legumes, whole grain bread, and olive oil characterize the Mediterranean diet. The emphasis is on a variety of minimally processed and, wherever possible, seasonally fresh and locally grown plant foods. Fresh fruit is taken as the typical daily dessert; sweets are consumed not more than a few times a week. Olive oil is used as the principal fat—shortening, margarine, butter, and other hard fats are rarely used. Total fat is about 30 to 35 percent of calories, with no more than 7 to 8 percent of it being saturated fat. Animal foods are eaten in moderation, with red meat used not more than a few times a month, poultry slightly more, and fish two to three times a week. Four or less eggs are used each week. Some dairy is eaten—primarily cheese and yogurt. Wine is consumed in moderation, normally with meals: about one to two glasses per day for men and one glass per day for women.

What does a very low-fat vegetarian diet look like?

A wide variety of vegetables, fruits, whole grains, and legumes are the basis of very low-fat vegetarian diets. Added fats of any kind, including oils, margarine, butter, shortening, oil-based salad dressings, and mayonnaise are almost totally avoided. Higher-fat plant foods such as nuts, seeds, avocados, and olives are totally eliminated or greatly restricted. The total fat content of the diet is usually less than 10 percent of calories with saturated fat generally about 2 percent. Some very low-fat vegetarian diets include small amounts of egg whites and nonfat milk products, while others are strictly vegan (no eggs and dairy products, as well as no meat).

diet had much less saturated fat and cholesterol, and had a far better balance of essential fats. (See pages 71-73.) By the end of two years, those eating the Mediterranean diet had an unprecedented 76 percent lower risk of dying of a heart attack or stroke.

Making Sense of the Dichotomy

How can it be that both of these eating patterns are so seemingly different, yet so effective in protecting against heart disease? First, while Mediterranean-style diets and very low-fat vegetarian diets contain very different amounts of total fat, they are remarkably similar in other ways. Both eating patterns are based on vegetables, legumes, whole grains, and fruits, and both provide abundant plant protein, fiber, vitamins, minerals, and other important compounds—all protective to heart health. Neither eating pattern is high in saturated fat, trans fatty acids (see page 40), cholesterol, or animal protein—all of which may promote heart disease. Their primary difference is that one program includes olive oil and higher-fat plant foods such as nuts, seeds, olives, and avocados. Obviously, these high-fat foods are not responsible for the detrimental effects often seen with other high-fat diets.

The Best of Both Worlds

There are advantages and disadvantages inherent in both very low-fat vegetarian diets and high-fat Mediterranean-style diets. When these are considered, one cannot help but imagine where we could be if we embraced the best of both diets and met somewhere in between! The World Health Organization (WHO) and the Food and Agriculture Organization (FAO) recommend an upper limit of 30 percent of calories from fat for most individuals and a healthy range of fat intake between 15 to 30 percent. Optimal fat intakes for people with type 2 diabetes fall very nicely into this range, with individual recommendations varying according to weight goals and calorie needs. However, it is extremely important to recognize that the amount of fat we eat is not as critical as the type of fat we eat.

Disease risk is more strongly associated with sources of fat than with the amount of fat in the diet. If the primary source of fat is whole plant foods (nuts, seeds, soy, avocados, and olives), one can expect to maintain excellent health eating a relatively high proportion of total calories as fat (i.e., 30% of calories). In contrast, when fat is derived from animal sources and processed fats (i.e., hydrogenated oils), adverse health consequences could be realized with relatively moderate total fat intakes.

Potential Problems with Very Low-Fat Diets

There are four potential problems with using very low-fat vegetarian diets for individuals with type 2 diabetes, all of which must be considered when putting together an optimal eating pattern.

1. *Very low-fat diets may provide insufficient long-chain omega-3 fatty acids, a type of polyunsaturated fat found in fish oil, flax seeds, walnuts, and green leafy vegetables. (See pages 71-75 for more information.)* This is no minor detail. Omega-3 fatty acids have been shown to provide significant protection against heart disease. They lower triglycerides, decrease blood-clotting tendency, and help to prevent irregular heart beat. These protective effects are especially important in people with type 2 diabetes, who often struggle with high triglycerides and who are at increased risk for heart disease. There is also solid evidence to suggest that omega-3 fatty acids may have beneficial effects on other diabetic complications, such as diabetic nerve damage and kidney damage. Very low-fat vegetarian diets (no added fat and limited fat-rich plant foods such as soy products, nuts, and seeds) generally provide only about 25 to 30 percent of the omega-3 fatty acids a person needs.

2. *The absorption of fat-soluble vitamins, minerals, and phytochemicals (health-promoting substances found in plant foods—see pages 55-59) may be compromised in very low-fat diets.* Studies indicate that there are some nutrients whose absorption is enhanced by moderate amounts of fat in the diet: fat-soluble vitamins (such as vitamin E, and substances called carotenoids, which form vitamin A), some minerals, and phytochemicals. Maximizing the absorption of these protective dietary constituents is especially important for people with chronic diseases such as diabetes.

3. *The overall nutritional value of the diet may be reduced when fat content is considered the highest priority in food selection.* Many individuals following very low-fat diets become highly "fat phobic," fanatically avoiding all foods that contain fat. In so doing, they may shun nutritious, whole plant foods such as nuts, seeds, avocados, olives, and even full-fat soy products such as tofu. These foods are among our richest sources of vitamin E and selenium (which protect against tissue damage), other trace minerals, and a host of protective phytochemicals (page 55), and have all been shown to be protective to health.

4. *Very low-fat, high-refined-carbohydrate diets can cause a drop in HDL cholesterol ("good cholesterol") and a rise in triglycerides.* Low HDL cholesterol and high triglycerides are associated with an increased risk for heart disease. However, these changes are generally only seen when the carbohydrates are derived from refined foods such as products based on white flour, or sugar-laden treats. When whole grains are used, changes in HDL and triglycerides are far less dramatic. In several studies, whole food diets that are high in carbohydrates have actually resulted in marked decreases in triglyc-

erides. HDL cholesterol may or may not fall with very high-carbohydrate diets. It is important to note that while we want to preserve or even increase HDL, if possible, a drop in HDL generally goes hand in hand with a total cholesterol reduction. This is because the primary function of HDL is the removal of excess cholesterol from the bloodstream; when there is less cholesterol to remove, there is less need for HDL cholesterol. Thus, while some decrease in HDL levels may occur, the drop in LDL is generally even greater, meaning an overall improvement in cholesterol levels. Relatively low HDL levels are seen in many societies that eat plant-based diets, and they are at very low risk for heart disease.

Potential Problems with High-Fat Diets

There are also potential problems to consider when using higher-fat diets for individuals with type 2 diabetes.

1. *High-fat diets may be linked to insulin resistance and/or impaired insulin secretion.* All high-fat diets cause insulin resistance when compared to high-carbohydrate diets; however, saturated fats appear to have the most negative effects on insulin action. Insulin secretion may also be impaired by high fat intake, with trans fatty acids causing the most problems. (See more on trans fats on pages 40-42.)

2. *High-fat diets can lead to obesity.* Ounce for ounce, fat provides more than double the calories of protein or carbohydrate. It also has less bulk, thus may promote overeating. In addition, dietary fat is stored as body fat more readily than carbohydrate or protein. Generally, where populations consume higher levels of fat, the incidence of obesity is greater (especially where people are sedentary) and the risk for several chronic diseases increases.

3. *High-fat diets can dilute nutrient density (the amount of nutrients per calorie of food), making it a challenge to meet recommended intakes for nutrients.* This is especially a concern for those who are attempting to lose weight and restricting calories. The problem is compounded when the main sources of fat are concentrated fats and oils such as vegetable oils, butter, margarine, and mayonnaise, and foods prepared or manufactured with these fats (as opposed to nuts, seeds, soy, avocados, and other whole foods). Refined fats and oils have no vitamins (except for vitamin E), minerals, protein, fiber, or other protective substances. (Unrefined oils contain small amounts.) When these fats and oils are abundant in the diet, it can be difficult to meet needs for nutrients that are often low to start with (such as calcium and magnesium).

4. High-fat diets may result in increased oxidative damage to body tissues.
Free radicals are reactive oxygen molecules containing one or more unpaired
electrons. (Most molecules are stable, containing only paired electrons.)
These electrons react quickly with other molecules, turning them into free
radicals, setting off a destructive chain of oxidative damage to tissues. (For
more on oxidation, see page 51-54.) Free radicals react mainly with unstable
fats, so people consuming large amounts of fat and few antioxidants from
plant foods could be more susceptible to oxidative damage. Oxidative stress
has been linked to numerous diseases, including heart disease, cancer, diabetes, arthritis, and neurological disorders.

Goal #2: Healthy Weight Promotion

The second major goal of diet therapy is promoting a healthy or desirable
body weight. Well over 80 percent of people with type 2 diabetes are overweight (some estimates are as high as 97 percent), with approximately 40
percent being obese. As body fat increases, so does insulin resistance. Being
overweight also contributes to high blood pressure and heart disease. Several
recent studies have demonstrated that weight loss in people with type 2 diabetes is associated with decreased insulin resistance, improved blood sugar
control, reduced blood cholesterol and triglyceride levels, and reduced blood
pressure. Clearly, achieving and maintaining a desirable body weight is one of
the most important aspects of diet therapy. It is fundamental to permanent
improvements in, and possibly reversal of, type 2 diabetes.

What type of diet best supports weight loss goals? Without a doubt,
whole foods, high-fiber, plant-based diets have the upper hand. Several important studies have demonstrated a positive connection between total fat intake
and body "fatness." Conversely, a number of recent studies have shown that
even with unrestricted quantities of low-fat, unprocessed plant foods (vegetables, fruits, whole grains, and beans), significant weight loss generally occurs.
Thus, for people with type 2 diabetes who are attempting to shed pounds, a
moderately low-fat diet, in the range of 20 to 25 percent calories from fat

> The importance of achieving and maintaining a healthy body weight cannot be
> overemphasized for overweight people with type 2 diabetes. Weight loss is
> fundamental to improvements in blood sugar control and absolutely essential to
> reversal of this disease.

makes good sense. (In this case a 2,200 calorie diet would contain 50 to 65 grams of fat a day.) This is halfway between a Mediterranean-style diet and the very low-fat vegetarian diet. To optimize essential fatty acids, mineral absorption, and overall nutritional quality of the diet, a limited amount of higher-fat plant foods such as nuts, seeds, olives, and avocados should be included. Small amounts of high-quality oils such as extra-virgin olive oil may also be used. (See chapter 4 for more detailed information on achieving a healthy body weight.) Of course, diet is only half of the weight loss equation— exercise is every bit as important.

Goal #3: Blood Sugar Control

The third and final goal of diet therapy is to achieve and maintain excellent control of blood sugar (glucose) levels. Poor blood sugar control increases the chance of damage to the eyes, kidneys, and nerves. To best promote blood sugar control, we can begin by looking at the specific dietary factors that affect it most. We need to consider both how much blood sugar increases and how rapidly it increases. The goal is to keep blood sugar from rising too high or too fast. Of course, we must recognize that there are also important nondietary contributors to blood sugar control, including exercise and stress management. (See chapter 8.) The dietary factors, which are thought to have the greatest impact on blood sugar control include

  1. Carbohydrates
  2. Fiber
  3. Fats
  4. Frequency of eating

> To best promote blood sugar control, we need to consider both how much sugar increases and how rapidly it increases.

Carbohydrates

Carbohydrates have the greatest impact on blood sugar levels. This is no big surprise as carbohydrates are simply sugars in various forms. Many people assume that "simple carbohydrates" (sugars) are the villains and that "complex carbohydrates" (starches) are far less damaging. This is not only a gross oversimplification, it is inaccurate. Simple carbohydrates are found in highly refined, nutrient-depleted foods like table sugar, but they are also found in highly nutritious whole foods like fruits and vegetables. Complex carbohydrates are found in heavily processed foods like white bread and pastries, but are also present in nutrient-dense foods such as wheat berries and beans. The old rudimentary view of simple versus complex carbohydrates becomes quite meaningless when considered in this context. Our glycemic (blood sugar) response to carbohydrates depends on many factors beyond whether they are in the form of sugars or starches. It is influenced by

1. *The number of grams of carbohydrate present.* The greater the carbohydrate content, the higher the blood sugar will rise.

2. *The type of sugar (glucose, fructose, sucrose, lactose).* Glucose causes a greater rise than sucrose (table sugar) or lactose (milk sugar), both of which cause a greater rise than fructose (fruit sugar). (See pages 43-46 for more details about various carbohydrates.)

3. *The kind of starch (amylose versus amylopectin).* Yes, there is more than one kind of starch! Amylopectin is broken down and absorbed more rapidly than amylose. Starchy foods contain different amounts of these two starches. For example, rice is higher than pasta in amylopectin, so it causes a greater rise in blood sugar.

4. *The amount and type of fiber present.* High-fiber diets can help to slow the absorption of carbohydrates. Soluble fiber slows the absorption even more than insoluble fiber. (For more information on types of fiber see pages 63-68.)

5. *The form of the food (cooked, raw, dry, liquid, paste, ground, or otherwise processed).* Food processing and cooking reduce particle size and increase the effect on blood sugar. Higher-density foods (foods containing less air) cause less of a blood sugar rise than lower-density foods (e.g., pasta causes less rise than bread).

6. *The presence of other components in the food or in foods eaten with the carbohydrate-rich food.* Fat and other food components slow digestion. For example, chocolate, rich in both sugar and fat, causes less of a rise in blood sugar than brown rice. (However, there are other reasons to choose brown rice over the chocolate!)

A tool called the *glycemic index (GI)* helps to give this information practical relevance. The GI is a way of classifying foods according to their effect on blood sugar. It is determined by feeding test foods in portions containing

50 grams of carbohydrates. Blood sugar levels are carefully measured over a three-hour period after eating the test food and a response curve is plotted, showing how high the levels got and how long they stayed that way. This is then compared to the curve of a standard reference food—usually glucose or white bread. The standard food is given a value of 100, and the test food value is expressed as a percent of how high and how long the reference food made blood sugar levels go up. The glycemic index of several foods is provided in table 2.1.

Glycemic index is not simply a measure of how fast sugar enters the bloodstream or how high the peak of the curve rises, as is commonly assumed. Rather, it is a measure of the area "under the curve," indicating that a food causing a wide but gentle blood sugar curve (gradual, long-lasting rise) can have the same glycemic index as a food causing a sharper spike (quick, large rise and fall). The more glucose that reaches the blood in the first three hours, the higher the GI will be. A quick rise and fall is less desirable for people with diabetes, because large peaks and valleys in blood sugar can increase the risk of complications. Thus, while the GI is a useful tool for people with diabetes, it is not perfect. It must be used with due consideration of other factors such as the overall nutritional value and composition of the food in question. Figure 2.1 provides an example of how two foods with identical glycemic indexes can have very different curve shapes, and different effects on health.

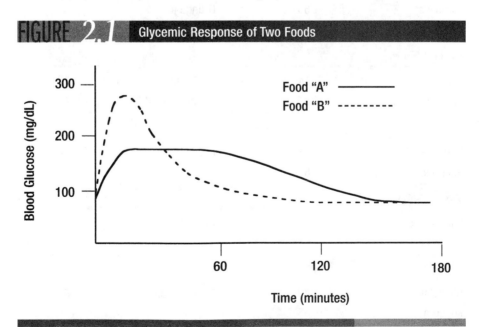

FIGURE 2.1 Glycemic Response of Two Foods

TABLE 2.1 — Glycemic Index (GI) of Selected Foods* (glucose = 100)

FOOD PRODUCT	GLYCEMIC INDEX	FOOD PRODUCT	GLYCEMIC INDEX
Grains			
Barley	25	Rye berries	34
Wheat berries	41	White spaghetti	41
All-bran cereal	42	Heavy grain breads	45
Cookies, oatmeal	55	Rice, brown	55
Rice, white	56	Oatmeal, all types	61
Whole-wheat bread	69	White bread	70
Cornflakes	84		
Vegetables			
Peas or corn, frozen	47-48	Sweet potatoes	54
Potatoes, boiled	56	Beets	64
Potatoes, mashed	70	Carrots	71
Fruits			
Grapefruit	25	Apples	36
Oranges	43	Bananas	53
Mangoes	55	Orange juice	57
Watermelon	72		
Legumes			
Peanuts	14	Soybeans	18
Most other legumes	26-38	Canned baked beans	48
Sugars			
Fructose	23	Lactose	46
Sucrose	65		
Dairy Products			
Milk, whole	27	Milk, skim	32
Ice cream	61		
Other			
Chocolate	49	Potato chips	54
Popcorn	55		

* Glycemic indexes provided in this table are adapted from average values provided in the International Tables of Glycemic Index (1995).

A newer tool, *glycemic load (GL)*, may actually be even better for assessing a food's overall impact on blood sugar than GI. Glycemic load is defined as the amount of carbohydrate in a food multiplied by the glycemic index. It provides a more meaningful measure of the glycemic burden of food because it takes into account the amount of carbohydrate eaten. The GL of a *small* quantity food with a *high* GI can be as great as a *larger* amount of food with a *low* GI. Although GL is generally less well recognized and used, diets with a high GL have been found to increase the risk of developing type 2 diabetes. They have also been associated with reduced HDL cholesterol levels ("good" cholesterol) and increased triglycerides.

Fiber

The effect of fiber on blood sugar has been the subject of considerable debate among researchers. For many years it has been recognized that fiber slows both carbohydrate absorption and a rise in blood sugar. However, the impact of fiber is relatively moderate unless the amount of fiber eaten is substantially above usual intakes. Most of the positive effects of fiber are due to soluble fiber. Research on fiber and glycemic control indicates that

- 10 to 20 grams of fiber a day has little impact on glycemic control. This is the amount of fiber consumed by the average North American.
- 20 to 35 grams of fiber a day provides some benefits to glycemic control, but less than previously expected. This is the amount of fiber typically recommended for good health.
- 35 to 50 grams or more of fiber a day has significant positive effects on glycemic control. Lacto-ovo vegetarians consume about 30 to 40 grams of fiber a day, and vegans consume 40 to 50 grams a day.

Lacto-ovo vegetarians: those who do not eat meat, poultry, or fish, but do use dairy products and eggs.

Vegans: those who do not use products of animal origin, including eggs, dairy foods, gelatin (made from the bones and connective tissue of animals), and honey (the product of bees).

Fats

Does the amount or type of fat in the diet influence blood sugar control? It seems like such an obvious question. After all, fats don't require insulin in order to be metabolized. Therefore, it makes sense that high-fat diets would be best for glycemic control—right? As you might have guessed, things are rarely that simple. Both the amount and type of fat in the diet may affect glucose tolerance and insulin sensitivity.

Amount of Fat

High-fat diets can reduce glucose tolerance by decreasing the ability of insulin to bind to insulin receptors, resulting in insulin resistance. They may also impair glucose transport, or the movement of glucose (the sugar in blood) into the cells. Studies have shown that high-fat diets increase insulin resistance when compared to whole food, high-carbohydrate diets. In addition, high-fat diets have been shown, in some studies, to accelerate the progression from impaired glucose tolerance to type 2 diabetes. So while fat doesn't cause the surge of insulin that carbohydrates do, excessive amounts of fat do appear to have a negative affect on glycemic control.

Type of Fat

As is the case for heart disease risk, it seems as though the type of fat may play an even bigger role in controlling blood sugar than the amount of fat. The type of fat in the diet affects the type of fat in the tissues, which may, in turn, affect the transfer of fluids through cell membranes and insulin function.

Saturated Fat

A high saturated fat intake has been associated with higher risk of glucose intolerance and higher fasting glucose and insulin levels. Higher proportions of saturated fats in body tissues have been associated with higher insulin levels, lower insulin sensitivity, and higher risk of developing type 2 diabetes.

Unsaturated Fat

Diets high in monounsaturated and polyunsaturated fats (such as olive oil and other vegetable oils) have been associated with a lower risk of type 2 diabetes and lower fasting blood sugar concentrations. In addition, higher proportions of long-chain polyunsaturated fats (EPA and DHA—see pages 71-75 for more information) in certain body tissues have been associated with better insulin sensitivity. Replacing saturated fat with monounsaturated fat appears to improve insulin sensitivity; however, some studies suggest that the favorable effect may be lost in individuals with very-high-fat diets (37 percent or more of calories as fat).

Trans Fatty Acids

Research on the effects of trans fatty acids on blood sugar control are very limited. Although there is some evidence that trans fatty acids increase insulin secretion, we can't make conclusions about its effects on glycemic control. However, there is reasonable evidence to suggest that trans fatty acids contribute to the risk of type 2 diabetes and massive amounts of evidence that they increase risk of heart disease.

THE BOTTOM LINE

Too much fat can have a negative impact on blood sugar control, as may excessive intakes of saturated fat. Once again, a plant-based diet containing moderate amounts of fat derived mainly from whole plant foods appears the most protective.

Frequency of Eating

Does it really matter if you eat twice a day or six times a day? Would nibbling all day improve your glycemic response? Fifty years ago research showed that increasing meal frequency could improve blood sugar control in people with type 1 diabetes. As a result, it was commonly suggested that people with diabetes eat several small meals over the course of the day. More recently, research on people with type 2 diabetes has provided evidence both for and against the value of eating more often.

On the pro side, one study looked at glycemic control in people given the identical diet but on one day the food was provided hourly as small snacks (nibbling diet), while on the next it was given as three meals and a snack. The nibbling diet resulted in significant improvements in glycemic control compared to the normal diet. A second study comparing the effects of two versus six meals per day found that with the higher meal frequency, swings in blood sugar were greatly reduced and peak blood sugar levels dropped.

On the con side, at least two major studies have shown little, if any, beneficial effects of more frequent meals. One group of researchers tested a three-versus nine-meal regime over a period of four weeks. This study did not note any real differences in glycemic control or insulin response. Another study compared three identical diets served with different frequencies. Only modest differences in overall blood glucose levels and insulin secretion were noted with the varying patterns.

So what's the verdict? While increasing meal frequency from the normal three meals a day to five to six meals a day may help to moderate blood sugar extremes and reduce insulin response, the evidence is not conclusive. However, having more frequent meals does not seem to harm glycemic control, providing it does not lead to weight gain. This is an important provision. Some experts believe that more frequent meals may mean higher caloric intakes, and this is a definite concern for people with type 2 diabetes. So, providing that your caloric intake is in keeping with your weight goals, and you are eating regular, balanced meals, the way you spread out your caloric intake throughout the day can be left to personal choice.

Food for Thought

For many years, people with type 2 diabetes believed they had been inflicted with a disease that was permanent and degenerative. The best that they figured they could hope for was good management. This, they thought, would include a daunting diet, complete with charts, scales, and special diabetic foods.

Today, reports of dramatic improvements, and even reversal, of type 2 diabetes are giving new hope to people with this disease. People are beginning to recognize that type 2 diabetes is not the result of an infection, bacteria, virus, or even a lack of insulin. It is the product of diet and lifestyle choices that cause the body to become resistant to insulin. It is not unreasonable to expect that with the appropriate changes, insulin function could be vastly improved or, in some cases, completely restored. The good news is that the diet that best supports these kinds of improvements is one that is based on simple, whole foods. The next chapters will guide you though the practical steps you need to take to construct a diet that works.

CHAPTER 3

Defeating Diabetes with Diet

B renda: My father used to tell me that he'd rather live 50 good years enjoying his cigarettes and potato chips than live 75 years having to forgo the freedom to do the things he so loved. Besides, he'd say, "I could be hit by a truck tomorrow." He taunted me with this line of reasoning, grinning and sticking out his belly as he'd walk by with all his goodies. It drove me nuts.

Not surprisingly, he didn't quite reach the age of fifty when the first stroke hit. He hadn't been to a doctor in about twenty years. When he arrived at the hospital, things were even worse than we anticipated—his blood pressure was 240/120, and his blood sugar was over 500 mg/dL (28 mmol/L). Needless to say, he was put on

insulin immediately. One of the tests he had was an angiogram. His blood ves-
sels were so plaque-ridden and damaged by years of smoking and eating fatty
foods that the doctor had a tough time getting the tubes through them—so
tough, in fact, that he punctured a tiny hole in my dad's aorta. This eventual-
ly led to major surgery so his blood vessels could be reinforced with grafts.
The doctors figured if he didn't stop smoking he'd live three months, and if he
did stop, he might have three years.

I will never forget sitting on his hospital bed and hearing him say, "I don't
want to die." It was scary. My dad always had the answers, no matter how
difficult the circumstances, but this time he was grasping. I think it was at this
point that he recognized the value of health. Unfortunately, for so many people,
it is only when health is snatched away that they fully appreciate its value.

You see, health cannot be bought or sold; it does not come in pills or
potions. It is the product of many years of wise choices. This is a revelation
that can be truly life changing. Thank goodness it was for my dad. He quit
smoking, started eating hot oatmeal in the morning instead of bacon and eggs,
and more vegetables and beans instead of burgers and chips. He began riding
his bike, roller blading, curling, and golfing. It has been twenty years since his
stroke, and he is doing far better than the doctors ever predicted. Unfortu-
nately, despite all his efforts, he will never completely regain the circulation in
his legs or erase the pain that comes when he walks uphill.

There is no doubt my father was right when he said "I could be hit by a
truck tomorrow," but I still don't think that it's a good excuse to walk out in
front of one. We don't have the final choice in how we die, but we do have a
choice in how we live. My hope for all those who choose to neglect their
health in the name of freedom is that they will come to understand that making
choices that support health is no sacrifice—it is a privilege to be treasured. Over
a century ago, the famous Swiss writer and philosopher Henri Frederick
Amiel said, "In health there is freedom, health is the first of all liberties." He
was a very wise man.

This chapter will assist you in a complete diet transformation. It will
move you from food choices that contribute to disease and suffering to those
that promote great health. It involves two very simple steps.

Step 1: Take out the trash
In other words, get rid of the foods that are most concentrated in the dietary
components that are damaging your health and contributing to your diabetic
condition. These foods are some of the most destructive.

- saturated fats
- trans fatty acids
- cholesterol
- refined carbohydrates
- excessive animal protein
- excessive salt
- excessive alcohol
- and oxidants (pro-oxidants)

Step 2: Pile on the protectors

Choose to eat the foods that are concentrated in protective dietary components. These are among the most effective.

- phytochemicals
- antioxidants
- fiber
- plant protein
- and essential fatty acids

STEP 1: TAKE OUT THE TRASH

You've probably heard the saying, "There are no good foods and no bad foods," and the slogan "All foods can fit." These have been key messages of national nutrition campaigns in both the U.S. and Canada. The idea, of course, is that any food can be a part of a nutritious diet if it is used in moderation. This line of reasoning makes complete sense and generally holds true if the bulk of the diet consists of healthful foods and the occasional treat is thrown in. But what happens when the lion's share of the diet consists of foods that provide little if anything to nourish and protect the human body? Disease happens—like heart disease and diabetes—diseases that have become epidemics in the affluent world. It is no mere coincidence that upwards of 70 percent of our population die of these sorts of lifestyle-induced diseases and that over 60 percent are overweight. The whole concept of not labeling foods good or bad serves more to justify the consumption of nutritionally depleted foods than to educate consumers about wise food choices.

It is hard to understand why so much of our nutrition education dollar is directed towards feel-good messages, when people so desperately need to learn how to make choices that promote health and prevent disease. Perhaps it has more to do with politics than nutrition. Major sponsors of large nutrition education campaigns have not traditionally been fruit, vegetable, whole grain, legume, or nut marketing boards. Not surprisingly, meat, dairy, confectionary, and soda pop industries are far better able to foot the bill. Could it be that the sponsoring organizations are more comfortable with campaigns that promote "everything in moderation" than they would be with those that encourage people to eat more beans and vegetables and less meat and processed foods? If one is honest about it, deep-fried pork rinds don't fit into a nutritious diet, no matter how you serve them.

There are foods and components of foods that are damaging to health, and others that are highly protective. If you take a good look at the "all-American meal," you'll begin to understand why we need to take a harder line where nutrition education is concerned. The average double cheeseburger, medium fries, and a medium cola provide a whopping 68 grams of fat (17 teaspoons), almost half of which are saturated; about 15 grams of trans fatty acids; and almost 150 mg of cholesterol. This meal is low in fiber (the only grain is refined), high in salt (about 1,200 mg), high in sugar (20 teaspoons sugar—all from the cola), high in animal protein, and lacking in protective phytochemicals. To top it off, the fries are often cooked in hydrogenated cottonseed oil—one of the most heavily pesticide-laden crops on the planet. And if that isn't enough, overcooking these foods can produce carcinogens, and undercooking may result in food poisoning, like the dreaded E-coli. It's time the all-American meal got the all-American boot.

Saturated Fat

As we saw in the previous chapter, saturated fats are generally considered bad fats. High levels of saturated fat are consistently linked with elevated blood cholesterol levels, heart disease, insulin resistance, and several forms of cancer. Most North Americans eat about 30 to 40 grams of saturated fat every day, about twice as much as is considered to be healthful. Animal products are the greatest sources of saturated fats in Western diets. Saturated fat is hard at room temperature. The harder the fat, the more saturated fat it contains. Milk fat is more than 60 percent saturated, beef fat about 40 percent, chicken fat about 30 percent, and fish fat 20 to 33 percent. That compares with plant fats that are about 6 to 25 percent saturated, most being in the 10 to 15 percent range.

The important exceptions are the tropical oils. Coconut fat is more than 85 percent saturated, palm kernel oil more than 80 percent, and palm oil about 50 percent. However, tropical oils are rarely a major part of any North American diet, accounting for less than 2 percent of the total fat. There are differing opinions about the health consequences of saturated fats in tropical oils. Some experts believe that they are every bit as damaging as saturated fats from animal sources; others feel that they are less damaging because they are packaged with fiber and protective phytochemicals, not cholesterol. Studies suggest that when moderate amounts of tropical oils are consumed as part of a high-fiber, low- or no-cholesterol, plant-based diet, judicious use of these fats does not increase heart attack risk. By contrast, adding tropical fats to a standard North American diet already containing excessive saturated fat and cholesterol may simply be adding fuel to the fire.

How much saturated fat should we eat? The WHO/FAO Diet and Diseases 2002 report* suggests optimal intakes should be no more than 7 percent of the total daily calorie intake for people with type 2 diabetes. What that means in terms of actual quantities depends on your energy needs. For those on reduced-calorie diets (1,400 to 1,800 calories per day), it would be no more than 11 to 14 grams of saturated fat per day, or about one-third of what most Americans eat. For those with greater energy needs (2,000 to 2,400 calories a day), a maximum of 16 to 19 grams of saturated fat would be recommended, or about half of what most Americans eat. Table 3.1 provides average total and saturated fat content of a variety of foods and the percent of the total fat in the food that is saturated.

After looking at table 3.1, it is easy to understand why certain foods have little place in a diet designed to prevent or treat disease. For example, let's say you are eating 1,600 calories a day and trying to stay within the recommended saturated fat limit of not more than 7 percent of calories (12 grams of saturated fat). If you choose to have a T-bone steak, you could eat 4 ounces (10 grams of saturated fat) and stay within your saturated fat limit, however, it would be very slim pickings for the rest of the day. Of course, if you opt for a 6-, 8-, or 12-ounce steak, you'd be way over the top.

On the other hand, if you skip the meat and stick to plant foods, you could eat all of the following foods and still come in under your goal of no more than 12 grams of saturated fat:

- 10 servings of fruits and vegetables
- 6 servings of whole grains
- 1 serving of beans
- 1 serving of tofu
- 1 ounce of nuts
- 1 ounce of seeds

*Joint World Health Organization (WHO)/Food and Agriculture Organization (FAO) of the United Nations Expert Consultation on Diet, Nutrition, and the Prevention of Chronic Diseases (2002)

TABLE 3.1	Saturated Fat Content of Various Foods**		
FOOD	**TOTAL FAT**	**SATURATED FAT**	**SATURATED FAT**
	(grams)	(grams)	(% of total fat)
Cheeseburger, double patty, 1	44.0	18.0	41%
Ribs, 3 oz. (85 g)	26.1	10.8	41%
Ice cream, regular, 1 cup (250 mL)	14.6	9.0	62%
Pork chops, 3 oz. (85 g)	21.1	7.9	37%
Steak, T-bone, 3 oz. (85 g)	18.8	7.4	39%
Fried chicken, 2 pieces	27.0	7.1	27%
French fries, large	31.0	6.5	21%
Extra-lean ground beef, 3.5 oz. (100 g)	16.3	6.4	40%
Cheese, cheddar, 1 oz. (28 g)	9.4	6.0	64%
Milkshake, 11 oz. serving (325 mL)	9.5	5.9	62%
Potato chips, 2 oz. (57 g)	19.6	5.2	27%
Milk, whole (regular), 1 cup (250 mL)	8.2	5.1	62%
Lard, 1 Tbsp. (15 mL)	12.8	5.0	39%
Pie, apple, 1 piece	19.4	4.7	24%
Avocados, 1 medium	30.0	4.5	15%
Eggs, 2, boiled	10.6	3.2	30%
Milk, 2%, 1 cup (250 mL)	4.7	2.9	62%
Baked chicken breast, 3 oz. (85 g)	7.7	2.1	28%
Fish, salmon, 3 oz. (85 g)	10.5	2.1	20%
Soy oil, 1 Tbsp. (15 mL)	13.6	1.9	14%
Olive oil, 1 Tbsp. (15 mL)	13.5	1.8	14%
Walnuts, 1 oz. (28 g)	18.5	1.7	9%
Ham, lean, 3 oz. (85 g)	4.9	1.6	33%
Sunflower seeds, 1 oz. (28 g)	14.1	1.5	11%
Sunflower oil, 1 Tbsp. (15 mL)	13.6	1.4	10%
Almonds, 1 oz. (28 g)	15.0	1.2	8%
Canola oil, 1 Tbsp. (15 mL)	14.0	1.0	7%
Flaxseeds, 1 oz. (28 g)	9.4	0.9	10%
Tofu, firm, ½ cup (125 mL)	5.6	0.81	14%
Olives, 10 large	4.7	0.6	13%
Garbanzo beans, 1 cup ckd (250 mL)	4.3	0.44	10%

FOOD	TOTAL FAT	SATURATED FAT	SATURATED FAT
	(grams)	(grams)	(% of total fat)
Fish, cod, 3 oz. (85 g)	0.75	0.2	20%
Whole grains,* 1 cup cooked (250 mL)	1.0	0.17	17%
Legumes,* 1 cup cooked (250 mL)	0.8	0.15	19%
Vegetables,* 1 cup cooked (250 mL)	0.3	0.05	17%
Lettuce, romaine, 2 cups (500 mL)	0.22	0.03	13%
Fruits,* 1 serving	0.2	0.02	10%

*most varieties
**From the USDA Nutrient Database.

How to calculate the percentage of saturated fat in your diet:

Information you need:

1. The total calories you are eating (TC)

2. The total grams of saturated fat in the food you eat (SF)

There are 9 calories in 1 gram of fat.

SF x 9 (the number of calories per gram of fat) = the total calories from the saturated fat in your foods

(SF ÷ TC) x 100 = Percent of calories from saturated fat.

Example:

calorie intake = 1,600 calories

saturated fat intake = 12 grams

12 grams x 9 calories per gram = 108 calories

108 calories ÷ 1,600 x 100 = 6.75% of calories from saturated fat

PRACTICAL POINTER

Limit your saturated fat intake to not more than 7 percent of total calories. If you use any flesh foods, opt for fish. If you use dairy products, stick to nonfat options. Use tropical fats in moderation, if consumed.

Trans Fatty Acids

Remember when saturated fats were first found to have unfavorable effects on health? Lard and tropical oils were in the doghouse. Responding to consumer demand, manufacturers hurried to find suitable replacements for the saturated fats used to make cookies, crackers, and other convenience products. The solution was something that sounded quite wonderful—"all vegetable fat" or "100% vegetable shortening." Through the process of hydrogenation (the addition of hydrogen under pressure), and the addition of flavorings, vegetable oils were made to look and taste like hard animal fats. Margarine was designed to replace butter and shortening to replace lard. Manufacturers were delighted because the new products were economical and very resistant to oxidation (e.g., they could sit on the store shelf for a long time). They also worked exceptionally well for deep-frying because of their high smoking point (the temperature at which fat begins to smoke, which degrades its quality). This allowed for fast, high-temperature cooking.

Consumers were pleased. They believed that they were making more nutritious choices without giving up taste or changing how these fats worked in baking or cooking. After all, how could anything made from vegetables be unhealthy? Unfortunately, when we extract the oil from a plant (leaving behind the vitamins, minerals, fiber, and phytochemicals), then force hydrogen into the oil to turn it into a solid fat, we are far removed from the original soybean or corn kernel, and from any healthful properties they may have once had. As a final blow, this process of hydrogenation changes the configuration of some of the nutritious unsaturated fats in the oil to a damaging form called "trans fatty acids." These fats are often completely ignored on food labels and are truly a hidden menace to health.

Approximately 90 percent of trans fatty acids in the food supply are produced by the hydrogenation of vegetable oils. The remaining 10 percent are formed naturally from bacterial fermentation within the intestinal tracts of ruminant animals (such as cows and sheep). Technically, trans fatty acids are still unsaturated fats, but unlike the usual form of unsaturated fats, which have a curved shape, trans fatty acids are straighter, more rigid molecules. As such, trans fatty acids act far more like saturated fats than like unsaturated fats.

For many years trans fatty acids were considered a relatively minor player in health and disease. There were two reasons for this. First, intakes of trans fatty acids are considerably less than intakes of saturated fat (2 to 4 percent of calories compared to 12 to 14 percent of calories). Second, studies showed that trans fatty acids increased total cholesterol levels only 80 percent as much as saturated fats. This figure was deceiving to say the least. While the impact on total cholesterol is not quite as high as it is with saturated fats, the overall damage to heart health is worse. Trans fatty acids not only raise total cholesterol, but they lower HDL cholesterol ("good cholesterol"), raise a particularly harmful form of LDL cholesterol ("bad cholesterol") called Lp (a), and potentially increase triglycerides. Gram for gram, the adverse effect of trans fatty acids is estimated to be two to four times greater than that of saturated fatty acids.

In a recent study of more than 84,000 women (The Nurses' Health Study), trans fatty acids were strongly associated with an increased risk of type 2 diabetes, while polyunsaturated fats were associated with a reduced risk. The researchers estimated that by replacing 2 percent of calories from trans fatty acids with polyunsaturated fat, risk for type 2 diabetes would fall by 40 percent.

The WHO/FAO Diet and Diseases 2002 report suggests intakes of trans fatty acids should be less than 1 percent of calories. For someone eating 1,600 calories a day, that amounts to no more than 1.8 grams of trans fatty acids.

In practical terms, that means avoiding or minimizing foods that contain hydrogenated fats or partially hydrogenated fats. They are quite simply bad

TABLE 3.2   Trans Fatty Acid Content of Selected Foods*

FOOD	TOTAL FAT (g)	TRANS FATTY ACIDS (g)
Microwave popcorn, 3.5 oz. (100 g)	25.0	7.5
French fries, large	23.7	5.0
Cookies, chocolate chip, 4	12.0	5.0
Donut, honey-glazed, 1	15.0	3.8
Shortening, 1 Tbsp. (15 mL)	14.0	3.7
Cake, yellow commercial with frosting, 1 piece	12.8	3.2
Margarine, hard, 1 Tbsp. (15 mL)	12.0	3.1
Crackers, snack, 8	7.0	2.6
Margarine, soft, 1 Tbsp. (15 mL)	12.0	1.4
Potato chips, 2 oz. (57 g)	19.6	1.1

*From the USDA Nutrient Database.

news. The most concentrated sources of trans fatty acids in the North American diet are crackers, cookies, granola bars, chips, and other snack foods, baked goods, margarine, shortening, and deep-fried foods. Trace amounts in breads, seasonings, and other products are not as much of a concern. (See table 3.2 for amounts of trans fatty acids in common foods.)

PRACTICAL POINTER

Avoid foods containing added hydrogenated or partially hydrogenated fat, especially when it is a primary ingredient or the predominant fat in a product. Avoid deep-fried fast foods. If you use margarine, select one that is nonhydrogenated. Read labels.

Cholesterol

Have you ever wondered how much cholesterol a bowl of cashews or a whole avocado has? The answer is none. Cholesterol is made by animals, not plants, so all animal foods contain cholesterol, while plant foods are all cholesterol-free. So next time you choose a particular brand of peanut butter, vegetable oil, or other plant-based food because it says "no cholesterol" on the label, realize it is just a sales gimmick.

Cholesterol is a waxy, fatlike sterol. It is an essential component of every body cell, used in the formation and maintenance of cell membranes, to make bile salts for digestion, and to produce steroid hormones, which include the sex hormones and some of the stress hormones. The human body manufactures about 800 to 1,000 mg of cholesterol each day, and there are no requirements for any additional cholesterol from food. There are several concerns about eating too much cholesterol because it can cause blood cholesterol levels to rise, increasing the risk of blood clots, heart attack, and stroke. For this reason, it is recommended that people with type 2 diabetes limit total cholesterol to less than 300 mg a day, and less than 200 mg a day if LDL cholesterol levels are greater than 100 mg/dL (2.6 mmol/L).

Plants also contain sterols called phytosterols ("phyto" means plant), which are most concentrated in higher-fat plants such as nuts, seeds, and avocados. Although they are chemically similar to cholesterol, they have been shown to exert significant beneficial effects. (See page 56.)

The most concentrated sources of cholesterol are organ meats and eggs. Contrary to what many people believe, there is little difference in the cholesterol content of meat, poultry, or fish, as cholesterol is stored primarily in muscle tissue. (See table 3.3 for the cholesterol content of some common foods.)

TABLE 3.3	Cholesterol Content of Common Foods*		
FOOD	**CHOLESTEROL (mg)**	**FOOD**	**CHOLESTEROL (mg)**
Sweetbreads (brain), 3 oz. (85 g)	1,800	Butter, 1 Tbsp. (15 mL)	30
Liver (poultry), 3 oz. (85 g)	570	Ice cream, 10% milk fat,	
Liver (beef), 3 oz. (85 g)	330	½ cup (125 mL)	30
Kidney, 3 oz. (85 g)	330	Hard cheese, 1 oz. (28 g)	30
Eggs, whole, 1	210	2% milk, 1 cup (250 mL)	20
Shrimp, 3 oz. (85 g)	165	1% milk, 1 cup (250 mL)	10
Veal, venison, 3 oz. (85 g)	100	Skim milk, 1 cup (250 mL)	5
Beef, pork, lamb, poultry, 3 oz. (85 g)	75	Nuts and seeds, any amount	0
Fish, most, 3 oz. (85 g)	50-75	Legumes, any amount	0
Milk, whole, 1 cup (250 mL)	35	Vegetables and fruits, any amount	0

*From the USDA Nutrient Database.

PRACTICAL POINTER

Limit intake of cholesterol-rich foods. Keep total cholesterol to less than 300 mg a day, and preferably under 200 mg a day.

Refined Carbohydrates

When we refine a kernel of wheat to produce white flour, we remove two things: the bran (where most of the fiber is) and the germ (the storehouse of nutrients including protein, vitamin E, vitamins, and minerals). What we are left with is endosperm, otherwise known as starch. In removing bran and wheat germ from a kernel of wheat, we squander some valuable resources. Lost are 95 percent of the phytochemicals, 90 percent of the fiber, and 75 percent of the vitamins and minerals. The white flour we are left with is used to prepare many favorite foods, like bread, pasta, cereals, crackers, pretzels, cookies, and other baked goods. Sometimes we add nutrients back to the flour before making these products in an effort to prevent nutritional deficiency diseases. This is called enrichment. The nutrients that are most often added back are the B vitamins thiamin, riboflavin, niacin, and folate, and the mineral iron. Unfortunately, none of the fiber or phytochemicals are added back, nor are many of the vitamins and minerals, like zinc, magnesium, chromium, manganese, selenium, copper, and vitamin E. So, although enrichment is desirable, it is a very distant second choice to leaving the grain intact. In North America more than 98 percent of all the flour we use is refined white flour.

Sugars, like white flour or white rice, are also refined carbohydrates. The key difference is that white flour is a starch or polysaccharide (a long chain of sugars bound together) and sugars are monosaccharides or disaccharides (mono, meaning a single sugar molecule and di, meaning two sugar molecules bound together). While most of us picture white table sugar when we hear the word "sugar," it is only one of several foods we use as sweeteners. Other common sugars include molasses, honey, corn syrup, maple syrup, brown sugar, invert sugar, dextrose, maltose, glucose, and fructose. Regular table sugar is made from either sugar beet or sugar cane and is 99.9 percent pure sucrose (a combination of two simple sugar molecules—glucose and fructose). Like other refined carbohydrates, it has been stripped of most of its valuable constituents, although to an even greater extent.

A hundred years ago people ate about 20 pounds (9 kg) of sugar a year or 6 teaspoons a day (30 mL). Today, we eat an average of about 78 pounds (35 kg) per year, 25 teaspoons per day (125 mL), or 22 percent of our total calories. A third of this sugar comes in the form of beverages, such as soda pop and fruit drinks. Our sugar intake has increased 27 percent between 1982 and 1996. Among the greatest contributors to this increase has been the super-sizing of soft drinks. Fifty years ago, a typical soft drink at a fast food restaurant contained 8 ounces (250 mL) of soda and 7 teaspoons of sugar (35 mL). Today, a typical mini- or child-size portion is 12 ounces (375 mL) and 10 teaspoons of sugar (50 mL), while a large 32-ounce (1 L) soft drink contains 27 teaspoons (135 mL) of sugar. The USDA recommends limiting added sugars (from packaged foods and the sugar bowl) to not more than 6 teaspoons (30 mL) a day for people on a 1,600-calorie diet, and 12 teaspoons (60 mL) a day for those on a 2,200 calorie diet. The WHO/FAO Diet and Disease 2003 report suggests limiting free sugars to less than 10 percent of calories. Don't forget that these limits were intended for nondiabetic individuals, thus it is possible that even lower intakes would be preferable for people with diabetes. For the sugar content of some common foods, see table 3.4.

TABLE 3.4	Sugar Content of Common Foods*
FOOD	**SUGAR TSP (ML)**
Mister Misty DQ Slush, 32 oz. (1 L)	28 tsp. (140 mL)
Fruitopia, strawberry, 20 oz. (625 mL)	18 tsp. (90 mL)
Orange soda, 12 oz. (375 mL)	13 tsp. (65 mL)
Cinnamon roll, 7.5 oz. (210 g)	12 tsp. (60 mL)
McDonald's vanilla shake, 20 oz. (625 mL)	12 tsp. (60 mL)
Pancake syrup, ¼ cup (60 mL)	10 tsp. (50 mL)
Pepsi, 12 oz. (375 mL)	10 tsp. (50 mL)
Low-fat fruit yogurt, 8 oz. (250 mL)	7 tsp. (35 mL)
Fruit "drink," 8 oz. (250 mL)	7 tsp. (35 mL)
Snickers bar, 1	6 tsp. (30 mL)
Kool-Aid, 8 oz. (250 mL)	6 tsp. (30 mL)
Pie, 1 slice	6 tsp. (30 mL)
Jell-O, ½ cup (125 mL)	5 tsp. (25 mL)
Hard candy, 1 oz. (28 g)	5 tsp. (25 mL)
Milk chocolate, 1 oz. (28 g)	4 tsp. (20 mL)
Baked beans, canned, 1 cup (250 mL)	4 tsp. (20 mL)
Dark chocolate, 1 oz. (28 g)	3½ tsp. (17.5 mL)
Presweetened cereal, 1 oz. (28 g)	3 tsp. (15 mL)

* From the USDA Nutrient Database.

At one time sugar was considered an absolute taboo for people with diabetes. This is no longer the case. The evidence from clinical studies shows that sugar does not increase glycemic response much more than the same number of calories from refined starches. As a result, experts have decided that people with diabetes can include sugar in their diet, in moderate amounts. While all this makes good sense, one important detail is too often overlooked. Although sugar appears to be not much worse than starch, it is *not* innocuous. Rather than giving sugar the stamp of approval, perhaps greater emphasis needs to be placed on cautioning against excessive use of refined carbohydrates in all forms (starches and sugars), including white flour products, white rice, *and* sugar. It is not that these refined starches and sugars are "poisonous." They are not, and they can be used prudently. On the other hand, they should never serve as dietary staples. Currently, as much as 70 percent of our energy intakes come from refined carbohydrate foods—foods rich in starch and sugar. This kind of intake results in disastrous consequences for health. Refined carbohydrates not only wreak havoc with glycemic control; they may adversely affect blood lipids (particularly triglycerides) and increase risk of other diseases. In addition, they manage to push out foods that nourish and protect us, and they provide little in the way of protective health benefits.

PRACTICAL POINTER

Refined carbohydrates, including both starches and sugars, should be minimized in the diet. A reasonable upper limit for people with diabetes is 2 servings per day.

Excessive Sodium

Which has more salt, an ounce (28 g) of potato chips or an ounce (28 g) of corn flakes? Surprise! The corn flakes contain almost double the salt of the chips. How can this be? Processed foods often have a lot of salt mixed into the raw ingredients to give them flavor. Potato chips and salted peanuts have salt on the outside of the food, making them taste salty, but it is not mixed into the raw ingredients.

The words salt and sodium are often used interchangeably, but actually sodium is a component of salt. Salt is 60 percent sodium and 40 percent chloride (hence, the chemical name sodium chloride). Salt is the most important source of sodium in the diet, although it is not the only source.

Sodium is a mineral essential to life. It is necessary for the maintenance of fluid balance, transmission of nerve impulses, and digestive processes. Nonetheless, most North Americans take in far more than is necessary, and in many cases these high intakes can contribute to health problems. Too much salt may increase the risk for stomach cancer, osteoporosis, and hypertension. People with type 2 diabetes are commonly affected by hypertension (estimates are as high as 60 percent or triple the nondiabetic population), increasing risk for heart attacks, stroke, and kidney disease. The link between sodium and blood pressure has been highly controversial. Part of the confusion stems from the fact that sodium does not affect everyone's blood pressure to the same degree—some people are very salt sensitive while others are not. Several studies have shown that a moderately reduced intake of salt causes no harm and may in fact do considerable good. Thus, a moderate salt intake is recommended for all North Americans.

The Dietary Recommended Intakes (DRIs) for sodium include a safe *minimum* intake of 500 milligrams a day, and an *upper limit* of 2,400 milligrams per day. However, the council also states that lowering sodium intake to 1,800 milligrams would probably be healthier. Twenty-four hundred milligrams equals about 6 grams or 1 teaspoon (5 mL) of salt. Average intakes are in the range of 2,400 to 7,000 mg per day.

Relatively small amounts of sodium occur naturally in foods (other than foods from the sea). About 75 percent of the salt we eat comes from processed foods, 20 percent from salt added at the table or in cooking, and 5 percent from sodium in unprocessed foods. The actual content of salt in foods is not as easy to surmise as one might imagine (see table 3.5). We can make a remarkable dent in our sodium intake just by knowing where it is hidden.

Salt-Smart Tips

1. Rely on whole foods as the foundation of your diet. If you use processed foods, keep your intake moderate.

2. Be aware of the sodium content of condiments and seasonings. Look for salt-free herb blends for cooking. Consider using salt substitutes such as potassium chloride instead of sodium chloride. If you are on medication, be sure to ask your doctor if salt substitutes are safe for you.

3. Read labels—sodium is almost always listed. Look for products that are low-salt or reduced-sodium.

4. Go lightly on salt added during cooking and at the table. Ask restaurant chefs to do the same. If you do add salt during cooking, add it near the end— you can get away with lesser amounts!

5. Use fresh or frozen vegetables and beans instead of canned, when possible. If you do use canned, rinsing the vegetables or beans reduces the salt content.

6. Limit your use of pickled products—they are soaked in salt!

TABLE 3.5 — Sodium Content of Common Foods*

FOOD	SODIUM CONTENT (MG)
Canned beans (no pork), 1 cup (250 mL)	1,008
Soup, 1 cup (250 mL)	1,000
Pickles, dill, 1 medium	833
Nachos with cheese, 6 to 8 nachos	815
Canned corn, 1 cup (250 mL)	572
Canned tomatoes, 1 cup (250 mL)	564
Macaroni and cheese, 1 cup (250 mL)	560
Pretzels, 1 oz. (28 g)	486
Cheese pizza, 1 slice	336
Soy sauce, 1 tsp. (5 mL)	302
Canned tuna, 3 oz. (85 g)	301
Cornflakes, 1 oz. (28 g)	300
Olives, 10 small	270
French fries, medium	265
Peanuts, salted	230
Gravy, packaged mix, ⅓ oz. (10 g)	218
Chocolate cake with frosting, 1 slice	213
Ketchup, 1 tablespoon (15 mL)	178
Cheese, 1 oz. (28 g)	175
Potato chips, 1 oz. (28 g)	160
Bread, whole-wheat, 1 slice	150
Cookies, oatmeal, 2	136
Crackers, Ritz ½ oz. (14 g)	109

* From the USDA Nutrient Database.

PRACTICAL POINTER

Keep sodium intake to less than 2,400 mg per day. Limit your use of processed foods, and moderate your intake of salty condiments. Go lightly with the salt shaker when cooking and at the table.

Excessive Alcohol

You are probably well aware that drinking too much alcohol is bad for your health. However, you may be a little less certain about the effects of moderate drinking. Research suggests that moderate alcohol intake may protect against heart disease and stroke (although it may increase triglycerides), while potentially increasing the risk of certain forms of cancer. For people with type 2 diabetes, studies show that, compared to abstinence and heavy drinking, moderate drinking may improve insulin sensitivity and may reduce the risk of developing diabetes. Before you crack open a bottle to celebrate the good news, you need to consider the negative aspects of excessive drinking.

Too much alcohol can cause serious problems for people with type 2 diabetes: less blood sugar control, rising triglycerides, and increased blood pressure. Chronic, excessive alcohol intake can also damage your pancreas.

Alcoholic beverages can have both hypo- and hyperglycemic effects in people with diabetes, depending on how much alcohol is consumed and whether or not it is taken with food. Using moderate amounts of alcohol with food has minimal effect on blood glucose or insulin levels. However, there is a risk of hypoglycemia when alcohol is taken on an empty stomach, especially for those on insulin.

The Dietary Guidelines for Americans recommends no more than two drinks per day for adult men and no more than one drink per day for adult women. This recommendation is also mentioned in the American Diabetic Association guidelines and considered acceptable for most people with type 2 diabetes. One drink is generally defined as a 5-ounce (155 mL) glass of wine, 1.5 ounces (45 mL) of distilled spirits, or 12 ounces (375 mL) of beer. Complete alcohol avoidance is advised for pregnant women and for people with certain medical conditions, such as pancreatitis or liver disease.

If you choose to drink, limit intake to not more than one drink a day for women and two drinks a day for men. To reduce the risk of a hypoglycemic reaction, have your drink with a meal or snack. Do not replace food with alcohol. If you are on medications, check to ensure that alcohol will not react with the drugs.

Excessive Animal Protein

In our culture, fat and carbohydrates are endlessly maligned, while protein seems beyond reproach. For people with diabetes, the value of protein is emphasized to an even greater extent than for the average healthy person.

It is little wonder that some of our most popular diets today are those that are loaded with protein. These diets propose protein intake at levels two to three times current recommended intakes. Many people adopt these high-protein regimens, delighted to discover a diet that justifies heavy meat consumption. By following one of these programs, you'd get about 150 grams of protein a day on a 2,000-calorie diet. While high protein intakes do not appear to adversely affect glycemic control, they can be damaging in other ways, especially when the protein comes from animal sources. Protein above 20 percent of calories is associated with declining kidney function—a significant concern for anyone with diabetes. Nearly one-third of individuals with diabetes will develop kidney problems or nephropathy. Once kidney problems start, they tend to follow a fairly predictable downhill course.

Several studies suggest that vegetable proteins may be less toxic than animal protein and more protective of kidney function. In addition to concerns about kidney function, excessive protein increases calcium losses in the urine, potentially contributing to osteoporosis. Animal protein also raises blood cholesterol levels about 5 percent, while plant protein lowers it about 5 percent. Foods rich in animal protein come packaged with saturated fat and cholesterol—two dietary constituents associated with elevated blood cholesterol levels and heart disease.

Despite all of these concerns, the prevailing attitude is that people with diabetes need a lot of protein, and the protein that is most often suggested is lean animal protein. For most people with type 2 diabetes, protein metabolism is normal, and no additional protein is required. However, some people with diabetes do need extra protein, although it is not for the reason that is commonly assumed. For many years, experts believed that protein slowed the absorption of carbohydrate, thus helping to improve blood sugar control. More recently, studies have shown that this is simply not the case. When you eat a specific amount of carbohydrate, say 50 grams, your blood sugar response is no different than if you eat the carbohydrate by itself or with protein. However, if the protein replaces some of the carbohydrates (e.g., instead of 50 grams of carbohydrates, you eat 40 grams of carbohydrates and 10 grams of protein), your blood sugar response will be lower. It is not lower because of the presence of protein, but rather because fewer carbohydrates were eaten.

So why would someone with diabetes require more protein? There are two common reasons. First, with poor blood sugar control (e.g., frequent high blood sugar or hyperglycemia), protein turnover increases (more protein is used). Second, the metabolism of people with diabetes is altered in a way that reduces the normal ability to spare or conserve protein during weight loss. Thus, people with diabetes who are losing weight may also need additional protein. The protein needs of people with poor blood sugar control or those who are losing weight are about 20 percent higher than they are for others, or about 1 gram per kilogram (kg) of body weight (1 kg = 2.2 pounds). For a person who weighs 80 kg (176 lb), that amounts to 80 grams of protein (16 grams above usual recommended intakes). For the protein content of several common foods, see table 3.6.

PRACTICAL POINTER

Aim for about 15 percent of total calories from protein, and no more than 20 percent. For most people that means about 60 to 90 grams of protein per day. Consider replacing most of the animal protein in your diet with plant protein.

Oxidants (Pro-Oxidants)

Oxygen is a basic necessity of life. It is also a highly reactive element; wherever oxygen is present, so is oxidation. There is simply no escaping it— oxidation is a part of numerous essential life processes, such as the release of energy within the mitochondria of cells, and the destruction of viruses and bacteria by the sentinel cells of the immune system. While a certain amount of oxidation is necessary and desirable, when it goes on unchecked it can be highly destructive to the human body.

TABLE 3.6   Protein Content of Common Foods*

FOOD	TOTAL PROTEIN (g)	% CALORIES FROM PROTEIN
Chicken, roasted, 3 oz. (85 g)	24.3	52%
Salmon, 3 oz. (85 g)	23.4	52%
T-bone steak, 3 oz. (85 g)	20.5	38%
Cod, 3 oz. (85 g)	19.4	92%
Pork chops, 3 oz. (85 g)	19.0	28%
Lentils, 1 cup (250 mL)	17.9	30%
Tofu, firm, ½ cup (125 mL)	17.4	40%
Ground beef, 3 oz. (85 g)	15.9	33%
Navy beans, 1 cup (250 mL)	15.8	24%
Tempeh, ½ cup (125 mL)	15.8	36%
Deli slices, 4 slices (2 oz./57 g)	15.0	85%
Vegan burger, 1	12.0	36%
Eggs, 2	11.0	35%
Textured soy, ¼ cup dry (60 mL)	11.0	56%
Veggie wieners, 1 (1½ oz./43 g)	10.0	85%
Pumpkin seeds, ¼ cup (60 mL)	8.5	17%
Sunflower seeds, ¼ cup (60 mL)	8.0	17%
Milk, 2%, 1 cup (250 mL)	8.0	25%
Almonds, ¼ cup (60 mL)	7.4	13%
Cheese, 1 oz. (28 g)	7.0	25%
Soymilk (selected varieties), 1 cup (250 mL)	5-8.0	19-21%
Spinach, 1 cup (250 mL) cooked	5.4	40%
Cashews, ¼ cup (60 mL)	5.2	10%
Corn, 1 cup (250 mL) cooked	5.2	11%
Broccoli, 1 cup (250 mL) cooked	4.6	35%
Mushrooms, 1 cup (250 mL) cooked	3.4	26%
Oats, ½ cup (125 mL) cooked	3.0	17%
Potatoes, 1 medium baked	2.8	8%
Bread, whole-wheat, 1 slice	2.7	15%
Rice, brown, ½ cup (125 mL) cooked	2.5	8%
Green beans, 1 cup (250 mL) cooked	2.4	18%
Cauliflower, 1 cup (250 mL) cooked	2.2	26%
Barley, ½ cup (125 mL) cooked	1.8	7%
Orange, 1 medium	1.2	7%
Banana, 1 medium	1.2	4%
Apple, 1 medium	0.3	1%

* From the USDA Nutrient Database

So what exactly is oxidation? It is a process by which fuel is burned for energy to operate the cellular machinery. As we saw on page 24, it is also the term that describes unstable oxygen molecules, or "free radicals," that react with other molecules in the cell, setting off potentially damaging chain reactions. Free radicals can attack fats, proteins, carbohydrates, DNA, and RNA. Unsaturated fats on cell membranes are primary targets, since the more unsaturated a fat is, the more unstable it is, and the more vulnerable to free radical reactions. Oxidants or "pro-oxidants" promote these reactions, while "antioxidants" inhibit them. When the supply of pro-oxidants exceeds the reserve of antioxidants, harmful effects may result from damage to important molecules, including cell membrane damage and even cell death. Oxidant damage appears to be one of the basic common mechanisms of disease and aging, and is profoundly important as an underlying cause of cancer, heart disease, damage to the immune system, and the degenerative diseases of aging.

People with diabetes appear to have higher levels of pro-oxidants in their systems, so are at an increased risk for oxidative damage. The danger of oxidative stress appears to be elevated by hyperglycemia. Thus, people with diabetes must take care to reduce their exposure to pro-oxidants in the environment and in their food, and ensure a sufficient intake of antioxidants. (See pages 59-60.)

> Free radical damage (caused by oxidants) contributes to aging and almost all degenerative diseases. People with diabetes may be at an increased risk for oxidative damage.

What poses the greatest risk of oxidative stress? Air pollution, tobacco smoke, radiation, sunlight, stress, toxic wastes, and various chemicals can all trigger the process. There are many dietary components that act as oxidants, including food contaminants such as pesticides, herbicides, fungicides, hormones, PCBs, DDT, and dioxins. Rancid fats are also highly destructive. The more unsaturated the fat, the more prone it is to oxidative damage. Free metals such as iron and copper can transform mildly reactive molecules into highly reactive oxygen radicals. Whole plant foods that provide the building blocks for anti-inflammatory messengers in the body are extraordinarily important if we are to tip the balance between pro-oxidants and antioxidants in our favor.

Minimizing damage from oxidants

While there are certain oxidants in the environment that are largely unavoidable, you can minimize your risk of oxidative damage by making wise food choices:

■ Select, store, and prepare your fats and high-fat foods carefully. Avoid cooking fats at very high temperatures. Do not allow oils to smoke when heated, and discard them if they do. Store highly unsaturated oils such as flaxseed oil and hempseed oil in the refrigerator. High-fat plant foods without their protective coating, such as nuts, seeds, and wheat germ, should also be kept refrigerated.

■ Minimize your exposure to pesticides, herbicides, fungicides, hormones, DDT, and dioxins, as well as PCBs and furans. Opt for organic foods when you can. Wash your produce well, whether it's organic or nonorganic. Limit intake of animal foods, especially fatty animal foods, as many of these chemicals are stored in the fat of animals. Dioxins and PCBs are particularly problematic. More than 90% of our exposure to dioxins comes from food. These chemicals concentrate as they move up the food chain. A small animal will ingest several polluted plants; then a larger animal will eat several of the smaller animals. The highest concentrations come in freshwater fish (especially from polluted waters), shellfish, and marine fish. Other significant sources include beef, pork, poultry, eggs, and dairy products. Plant foods contain very low levels of dioxins. Like other animals, humans store these chemicals in their fat.

■ Eat sufficient, but not excessive, amounts of iron and copper. These metals are usually attached to proteins or stored in tissues, but when they are "free" in the blood, they can act as powerful oxidants. As iron stores rise, free iron also increases. Excessive iron stores are far more common in meat eaters than in vegetarians, due to the high levels of heme (blood) iron in animal flesh. Heme iron in the diet is absorbed without regulation, as opposed to the naturally chelated iron occurring in plant foods, for which there are normal absorption controls present.

STEP 2 – PILE ON THE PROTECTORS

Many people assume that once they get rid of the worst offenders, like saturated fat and cholesterol, there is nothing more they can do to further improve their diet. They are mistaken. While getting rid of unhealthy foods is an extremely important first step, it is only half the battle. Fortunately, the other half is much more pleasant—adding a wide variety of delightfully delicious and nutritious foods. Begin by building a solid foundation of whole plant foods—foods that shift the balance away from harmful components that promote disease toward those constituents that will nourish and protect you. The old saying "You are what you eat" is more accurate than you may ever have imagined. Every single cell of your body is derived from the food you consume. Why would you choose to build these cells out of junk? The section that follows covers each of the primary protectors in the diet. Pay close attention, for these are your greatest allies.

Phytochemicals

People have known for a very long time that vegetables, fruits, whole grains, legumes, nuts, and seeds are healthful foods. Experts presumed that the substances that made these foods so good for you were vitamins, minerals, and fiber. Of course they were right, but only partly so. Over the past couple of decades, scientists have discovered a whole new arsenal of protective compounds packaged within every whole plant food. Collectively these are called phytochemicals. Phytochemicals are natural substances that regulate growth, defend against attacks by insects or fungi, and provide flavor, color, texture, and odor to plants. Luckily for us, when we eat plants, these powerful little protectors go to work on our behalf, and their potential for human health is simply remarkable.

To begin, many phytochemicals are strong antioxidants (see pages 59-60), quenching destructive free radicals. Others have tremendous anticancer activity, blocking tumor formation, reducing cell proliferation, and inducing enzyme systems that help rid the body of potent carcinogens. Phytochemicals also protect against cardiovascular disease by helping to reduce the formation of cholesterol, lower blood pressure, decrease blood cholesterol levels and platelet stickiness, reduce blood clot formation, open blood vessels, and decrease damage to blood vessel walls. A special group of phytochemicals, called phytoestrogens or plant estrogens, attach to estrogen receptor sites, but are only about 0.1 to 0.2 percent as potent as the primary human form of estrogen, estradiol. When estrogen levels are high, phytoestrogens may reduce the harmful effects of human estrogen by binding to receptor sites, crowding out human estrogen. There is some evidence this action may protect against hormone-related cancers. When estrogen levels are low, the weak estrogens may provide enough estrogenic activity to provide protection against diseases such as osteoporosis and heart disease.

Another important group of phytochemicals is called phytosterols or plant sterols. These compounds are structurally similar to cholesterol, but with remarkably different effects on the body. Plant sterols appear to compete with dietary cholesterol, reducing its absorption from the gut. Studies have suggested that sterols cut blood cholesterol levels, inhibit breast, prostate, and colon cancer cell growth, and reduce inflammation. As a bonus for people with diabetes, they also appear to help improve blood sugar control. Plant sterols are present in nuts, seeds, vegetable oils, grains, legumes, green leafy vegetables, and other plants. The average Western diet contains between 180 and 410 mg of plant sterols a day, while a diet that is primarily plant based contains closer to 600 to 800 mg a day.

The list of significant beneficial activities of phytochemicals goes on: immune-enhancing, anti-inflammatory, antiviral, antibacterial, antifungal, anti-yeast, and anti–motion sickness. Yet, remarkably, we do not routinely measure these important secondary nutrients in foods, and the agricultural market favors size and external appearance more than the nutritional quality of our produce. This is another area where organic foods may be superior. Grown on soils with intact microflora, the plants themselves are better nourished and, at least in theory, will contain more protective phytochemicals. While it may all seem a little overwhelming, just keep in mind that loading up on foods rich in phytochemicals is one of the very best ways that people with type 2 diabetes, with their inherently increased levels of oxidative stress, can protect themselves.

Which foods are the most efficient phytochemical factories? Vegetables and fruits stand out as being particularly noteworthy, although legumes, grains, nuts, and seeds are also excellent sources. Choosing a wide variety of colorful, whole plant foods is your key to a phytochemical-rich diet. There are, of course, certain foods that can transform your diet into a tremendous phytochemical feast. Among the most outstanding are dark greens (such as kale, collards, and spinach), crucifers (like broccoli and broccoli sprouts), garlic, tomatoes, blueberries, citrus fruits, flaxseeds, and soybeans. Let's take a look at some of the most impressive among these.

Phytochemical Superstars

■ KALE. Found to have the greatest antioxidant activity when rated against nineteen other vegetables, kale is rich in lutein (see page 61), a phytochemical that protects the eyes from macular degeneration, a major concern for people with diabetes and the leading cause of blindness in North America. It is also high in beta-carotene (antioxidant), indoles (help eliminate toxic compounds), sulforaphanes (anticarcinogens), and quercetins (anti-inflammatory agents).

■ BROCCOLI. With a similar complement of phytochemicals as kale, broccoli is also noted for its indole content (helping to shift estrogen production to a less potent form, a protective factor relative to hormone-related cancers). Interestingly, scientists have discovered that broccoli sprouts contain anywhere from ten to one hundred times more sulforaphane than broccoli, comparing weight for weight.

■ GARLIC. With a unique phytochemical makeup, garlic is loaded with allium compounds. These phytochemicals help to lower blood pressure, reduce the stickiness of blood cells, dilate blood vessels, and destroy cancer cells. Allium compounds also have immune-stimulating, antibacterial, antifungal, antiyeast, and antiasthmatic activity. It is little wonder that Hippocrates used garlic to treat infections and pneumonia!

■ TOMATOES. Tomatoes get their red color from the exceptional amount of lycopene they contain. Lycopene has strong antioxidant properties, and several studies have suggested that it may be effective in protecting against prostate cancer and/or slowing the growth of prostate tumors. As well, there is some compelling evidence that lycopene is a powerful protector against the development of artery and heart disease.

■ BLUEBERRIES. Thought to be one of the most protective foods on the planet, blueberries offer a lot of surprises. In a study by the USDA's Center for Aging at Tufts University, the oxygen radical absorbance capacity, or ORAC (ability to quench free radicals), of over forty vegetables and fruits was measured. Of all the foods, blueberries came out on top—even above all of the vegetables! Indeed it had five times the ORAC of most other fruits and vegetables. The primary active component in blueberries is a phenolic compound and powerful antioxidant called anthocyanin. This substance gives blueberries their rich blue color. (Deep shades of blue, purple, and red come from anthocyanin—great sources also include plums, deep purple grapes, and other berries.) Blueberries contain several other phenolic compounds, including flavonols and phenolic acids. In addition to their antioxidant activity, blueberries have been found to protect against urinary tract infections, improve "tired eyes," and possibly reduce the overall effects of aging through their potent antioxidant activity.

■ CITRUS FRUITS. Oranges, grapefruits, lemons, and limes contain not only vitamin C and folic acid, but a wonderful array of phytochemicals. A single orange contains over 170 different phytochemicals, including 60 flavonoids, 40 limonoids, and 20 carotenoids. (See more on these on pages 60-61.) Flavonoids are strong antioxidants with significant anticancer and anti–cardiovascular disease activity, while limonoids help to reduce cholesterol levels and stimulate detoxifying enzymes.

■ SOYBEANS. These beans provide a rich plant source of protein and plant sterols, as well as phytoestrogens such as lignans and isoflavones. The principle isoflavones in soy are genestein and daidzein. These isoflavones are powerful antioxidants and very effective inhibitors of the tyrosine kinase enzyme—a potent tumor promoter. Research suggests that isoflavones may provide protection against heart disease, certain forms of cancer, and osteoporosis. Some evidence also indicates that they may preserve cognitive function. While much press has been given to the potential for soy to ameliorate symptoms of menopause, results have been mixed. If it does provide benefit, it appears to be minimal.

■ FLAXSEEDS. The champions of the nut and seed world, flaxseeds are our richest known source of lignans (potent anticarcinogens), with over 100 times the lignans of most other plant foods. They also boast the highest alpha-linolenic acid content of any food—57 percent of the fat in flaxseeds is omega-3 fatty acids. Omega-3 fatty acids fight cancer and cardiovascular disease. Like other nuts and seeds, flaxseeds also contain flavonoids, phenolic acids, phytic acids, and tocotrienols (a type of vitamin E).

■ GREEN TEA. With its polyphenol and catechin content, green tea is an up-and-coming phytochemical superstar. It is especially rich in epigallocatechin gallate, a potent anticarcinogen and powerful antioxidant.

It is important to note that refining foods can dramatically diminish phytochemical content. (Recall that refining a grain of wheat removes 95 percent of the phytochemicals.) While many people assume that cooking will damage phytochemicals, that is not necessarily so. In many cases cooking actually increases the availability of phytochemicals. For example, lycopene is far better absorbed from cooked tomatoes than from raw tomatoes, especially when olive oil (or other cooking oil) is used in the recipe. Cooking can also alter the structure of phytochemicals, resulting in very different health effects. For example, when garlic is cooked in water, vinyldithiins (antiasthmatics) are produced, while when cooked in oil, ajoenes (inhibitors of chemicals that increase inflammation and blood pressure) are formed. There is little question that if you want to maximize phytochemicals in your diet, it is best to include a variety of both raw and cooked foods.

Many people wonder if they can just pop a pill to get their phytochemicals. For example, many multivitamins now contain lutein as a secondary micronutrient. For a host of reasons, it looks like we are much better off eating the whole food than simply relying on an extract. Studies looking at the effects of single phytochemicals have been rather mixed, and some downright discouraging. A case in point is beta-carotene. There is solid evidence to indicate that a diet rich in beta-carotene and other carotenoids protects against lung cancer. However, used as a supplement in two large trials, beta-carotene actually increased risk. One of the reasons for this may be that phytochemicals often work synergistically with one another, and the collaborative action of two or more chemicals is sometimes needed to produce the desired effect. At this time, we just do not know enough about the complicated interactions of these dietary components to be confident about turning them into pills. Besides, whole foods come packaged with fiber, vitamins, minerals, plant sterols, and other protective components, and they are infinitely more pleasurable to consume!

PRACTICAL POINTER

To increase the phytochemical content of your diet in a safe and effective manner, increase the quantity, color, and variety of whole plant foods eaten each day. Aim for at least seven servings of vegetables and fruits each day.

Antioxidants

While many consumers have never even heard of phytochemicals, most are quite familiar with antioxidants. It is common knowledge that antioxidants are highly protective dietary components, always ready to do battle with destructive free radicals. Antioxidants provide a defense force that has been shown to diminish the oxidative stress associated with almost every disease process known. For people with diabetes, there is some convincing evidence that they may even reduce the risk of complications, including blindness, kidney failure, amputation, and ultimately death. In a mixed study including people both with and without diabetes, patients with poor blood sugar control and early signs of complications had depleted their store of antioxidants. The association between high blood sugar and low antioxidant levels was striking. The ability to defend against free radical attack was approximately half in people with poorly controlled diabetes and early signs of complications as it was in individuals without diabetes. There is definitely good reason to pay close attention to antioxidants and attempt to optimize them in your diet.

Antioxidants come from two places—internal production and external intake. Everyone produces antioxidant enzymes such as superoxide dismutase, catalase, and glutathione peroxidase. These enzymatic antioxidants need to partner with certain mineral "cofactors" in our food to perform their radical scavenging action. The best recognized of these cofactors is selenium, although manganese, zinc, copper, and iron are also required by some enzymes. The most well-recognized antioxidants in our food supply are vitamins C and E, phytochemicals, and carotenoids. Other antioxidants that appear to be especially important for people with diabetes are glutathione, taurine, and alpha-lipoic acid.

Carotenoids

Carotenoids are yellow, orange, and red pigments found in plants, including dark green vegetables. (Chlorophyll masks the brightly colored pigments.) Plants make about six hundred different carotenoids, and about 10 percent of these can be converted to vitamin A in our bodies. Carrots, sweet potatoes, squash, and other vitamin A rich plant foods do not actually contain any active vitamin A, but rather these pro–vitamin A carotenoids. Different carotenoids have very different effects on disease. The most well-recognized carotenoid is beta-carotene, which is our most important plant source of vitamin A; others are alpha-carotene, gamma-carotene, canthaxanthin, cryptoxanthin, lycopene, lutein, and zeaxanthin. In addition to vitamin-like activity, carotenoids are antioxidants—efficient free radical scavengers.

The active form of vitamin A, which is found in animal foods, is a very poor antioxidant. While carotenoids in foods have been found to offer protection against cancer, heart disease, and type 2 diabetes, supplements do not appear to provide similar benefits. Researchers speculate that this is because of the variety of carotenoids and other protective compounds in plants that work together to provide beneficial effects.

Two carotenoids of particular interest to people with diabetes are lutein and zeaxanthin. These antioxidants have been shown to be associated with a reduced risk of macular degeneration and cataracts. As an antioxidant, lutein is estimated to be ten times more effective than vitamin E. Lutein and zeaxanthin are yellow pigments that filter out harmful ultraviolet and blue light known to cause free radical damage to the eyes. The best food sources of lutein are dark greens like spinach, broccoli, and kale, and other plant foods such as squash, corn, and peas. Zeaxanthin is concentrated in dark greens, corn, red peppers, oranges, mangoes, papayas, peaches, prunes, apricots, and melons.

It is important to note that dietary fat is important for the absorption of carotenoids. In one study, adding 4 teaspoons (20 mL) of olive oil to a diet containing 7 percent of calories from fat (basically a no-added-fat diet) increased the absorption of beta-carotene by five times. Fortunately, the amount of fat needed to maximize absorption is only about 20 percent of your daily calories. So next time you pile your plate high with dark leafy greens, tomatoes, carrots, and red peppers, don't feel guilty about topping it with a delicious dressing with extra-virgin olive oil instead of the fat-free, water-based chemical concoctions so many people view as the most nutritious choice.

Vitamin C

Vitamin C is a powerful water-soluble antioxidant, neutralizing potentially harmful reactions in the blood and the fluid both inside and surrounding cells. For people with diabetes, vitamin C appears to protect against impaired glucose tolerance, and possibly also against complications of diabetes, particularly eye damage.

A number of small studies have reported that people with type 2 diabetes have reduced vitamin C levels when compared to those without diabetes. This may be due to increased vitamin C excretion in people with diabetes. Overall, research suggests that dietary vitamin C may have a significant positive impact on both diabetes risk and management.

There is still considerable controversy about whether or not vitamin C supplements are useful for people with type 2 diabetes. Some experts believe that vitamin C intakes of approximately 200 mg per day are sufficient, and best obtained by eating several servings of vegetables and fruits rich in vitamin C each day. Others believe that people with type 2 diabetes are justified in taking supplemental vitamin C in the range of 1,000 to 2,000 mg per day.

The one thing that most experts agree on is that the RDA (recommended dietary allowance) for vitamin C (75 mg per day for women and 90 mg per day for men) is not sufficient for people with type 2 diabetes.

If you decide to take supplemental vitamin C, be aware that high doses can cause stomach irritation, nausea, and diarrhea. It can also reduce the effectiveness of certain diabetes medications, so check with your doctor before you begin. Vitamin C is best taken in at least two divided doses daily. If you are sensitive to acid, take a buffered form of vitamin C.

Vitamin E

While it is relatively easy to get plenty of carotenoids and vitamin C from foods, meeting needs for vitamin E is considerably more challenging. The average North American consumes only about half of the recommended 15 mg per day of vitamin E. (This amount is equal to 22 IUs of natural vitamin E [d-alpha-tocopherol] or 33 IUs of synthetic vitamin E [dl-alpha-tocopherol]). Among the most widely recognized of all antioxidant nutrients, vitamin E serves as an important bodyguard by sacrificing itself in order to protect fat and fat-soluble substances, such as vitamin A, from the ravages of free radicals. It stabilizes cell membranes, protects white blood cells, increases blood flow, and appears to protect against blood vessel damage to the eyes and kidneys. Some studies suggest that vitamin E may also help insulin work better.

The most concentrated sources of vitamin E are nuts, seeds, wheat germ, whole grains, leafy greens, broccoli, avocado, and vegetable oils. (Cold-pressed, unrefined oils have higher levels than refined oils.) A variety of vitamin E–rich foods should be eaten daily. If vegetable oils are used, avoid high heat (e.g., deep frying) as this can destroy vitamin E. There is some evidence suggesting that vitamin E supplements may be beneficial for people with type 2 diabetes. If you choose to take a vitamin E supplement, opt for a natural source (d-alpha-tocopherol or a mixture of tocopherols and tocotrienols). Based on a variety of studies, reasonable intakes would be in the range of 400 to 1,000 mg per day.

Glutathione

Glutathione is a vital part of our body's antioxidant defense system. It is manufactured by the body but also naturally occurs in several fruits and vegetables. This powerful protector has an amazing range of activities. Glutathione plays a key role in immune function, DNA repair, and the removal of toxic chemicals from the body. It also recycles vitamins C and E back to their active forms.

In people with diabetes (and anyone of advanced age), glutathione levels in the lens of the eye decrease, and this is believed to contribute to the development of cataracts. Glutathione supplements are ineffective, because glutathione is not efficiently absorbed by the intestinal tract. Experts believe that the best way to increase glutathione levels is to support the body's synthesis of it using alpha-lipoic acid (see page 177), vitamins C, E, B_6, and riboflavin, and the minerals copper and selenium.

PRACTICAL POINTER

The most important thing you can do to maximize the antioxidants in your diet is to increase your intake of a variety of colorful, whole plant foods—especially vegetables and fruits. Recommended intakes are five to ten servings per day, although a range of eight servings or more seems to offer even greater benefits. If you decide to use antioxidant supplements, be sure to discuss your choices with your doctor, as there are supplement-drug interactions that need to be considered. (For example, certain antioxidants can reduce the effectiveness of the cholesterol-lowering medication Zocor.)

Fiber

Fiber is the part of plants that cannot be digested by humans. All plant foods contain fiber—it is what gives them their structure. On the other hand, animals get structure from bones, so animal products like meat and dairy products are fiber-free. Fiber is often divided into two categories based on whether or not it dissolves in water. Structural fibers such as celluloses, some hemicelluloses, and lignins are insoluble. Wheat bran is an example of a food rich in insoluble fiber. When it is mixed with water, it absorbs the water, but does not dissolve or become gluey. Almost all whole plant foods are good sources of insoluble fiber. Gel-forming fibers such as pectins, gums, and mucilages are soluble. Oat bran is a rich source of soluble fiber. When mixed with water, it becomes sticky. Other good sources of soluble fiber include beans, peas, several fruits, barley, flaxseeds, some vegetables, and psyllium (used in some cereals and bulk-fiber laxatives). Most plant foods contain a

TABLE 3.7 — Fiber Content of Selected Foods

AMOUNT OF FIBER (ROUNDED TO THE NEAREST GRAM)

FOOD/SERVING SIZE

Ultra High-Fiber Foods (12 to 20 grams)

Legumes, most, 1 cup (250 mL) cooked

Green peas, cooked, 1 cup (250 mL)

High-fiber bran cereals (All Bran, Bran Buds with Psyllium), ½ cup (125 mL)

Very High-Fiber Foods (8 to 11 grams)

Legumes (lima beans, soybeans, black-eyed peas), 1 cup (250 mL) cooked

Grains (bulgar, buckwheat groats), 1 cup (250 mL) cooked

Dried fruits, 4 figs or pears, 7 peaches, 20 apricots

Pea soup, 1 cup (250 mL)

Cereals (Raisin Bran and other bran-enriched cereals), 1 cup (250 mL)

Berries (raspberries, blackberries), 1 cup (250 mL)

High-Fiber Foods (5 to 7 grams)

Grains (barley, cornmeal, whole-wheat pasta, oat bran), 1 cup (250 mL) cooked

Cereal, whole grain (Shredded Wheat), 1 cup (250 mL)

Cereal (Grape Nuts, granola), ½ cup (125 mL)

Bread, high-fiber whole grain, 2 slices

Potatoes, regular or sweet, 1 medium, baked

Vegetables (broccoli, Brussels sprouts, squash, eggplant, okra, dark greens, parsnips,
    carrots), 1 cup (250 mL) cooked

Artichoke, 1 medium

Berries (strawberries, blueberries), 1 cup (250 mL) fresh

Fruit (papayas, Asian pears, avocado), 1 medium

Flaxseeds, ground, 2 Tbsp. (30 mL)

Moderate-Fiber Foods (2 to 4 grams)

Grains (oats, millet, brown rice), 1 cup (250 mL) cooked

Pasta, white, 1 cup (250 mL) cooked

Bread, whole grain,* 2 slices

Fruit, most, 1 medium, 2 small, or 1 cup (250 mL)

Vegetables, (cabbage, cauliflower, green beans, asparagus, mushrooms, turnips, peppers, leeks, celery), 1 cup (250 mL) cooked, 1-2 cups (250-500 mL) raw

Nuts and seeds, most, ¼ cup (60 mL)

Popcorn, 3 cups (750 mL)

Low-Fiber Foods (1 gram or less)

Refined grains (white rice, Cream of Wheat cereal), 1 cup (250 mL) cooked

White bread, 2 slices

Baked white flour products (crackers, cookies, cakes, pastries, etc.), 1 serving

Cereals (Cornflakes, Rice Krispies, and other refined grain cereals*), 1 cup (250 mL)

Fruits (melon), 1 cup (250 mL)

Fruit juice, all varieties, 1 cup (250 mL)

Vegetables (iceberg or Bib lettuce), 1 cup (250 mL)

Potato chips, 1 oz. (28 g)

Candies, 1 serving

Fiber-Free Foods (zero fiber)

Meat, poultry, fish

Eggs

Milk, cheese, ice cream, and other dairy products

Fats and oils

* Read package labels for exact fiber content.

mixture of insoluble and soluble fiber, but generally contain far more insoluble fiber.

Both soluble and insoluble fiber are valuable to health. Among the most well-recognized benefits of fiber is keeping our gastrointestinal system clean and healthy. This effect comes largely from insoluble fiber, which adds bulk to the stools and ensures that foods pass quickly and easily through the intestinal tract. Soluble fiber is especially valuable for people with type 2 diabetes, because it helps to control blood sugar levels and reduce blood cholesterol. Few experts would disagree that fiber helps to protect us against almost every major chronic disease plaguing the Western world, including type 2 diabetes, heart disease, some forms of cancer, gastrointestinal diseases, hypoglycemia, and obesity. In order get your intake up in the 35 to 50 gram range, you need to aim for at least 10 to 12 grams of fiber per meal and another 4 to 5 grams with each snack (assuming one to two snacks per day). For ideas on how to pack fiber into your diet, check out the menu plans on pages 110-117. For a list of fiber in foods, see table 3.7 on the previous two pages.

People often have two concerns that arise when dietary fiber is raised to the extent recommended here.

1. Can too much fiber be harmful?

2. Won't eating this much fiber cause a lot of gas?

Can Too Much Fiber Be Harmful?

Yes—it is possible to get too much of a good thing! Although not generally a concern, excessive fiber can reduce the absorption of certain minerals such as calcium, iron, and zinc. The World Health Organization recommends an upper limit of 54 grams of fiber per day based on mineral balance. As a general rule, eating a wide variety of whole plant foods will not result in excessive intakes of fiber. It is important to note, however, that problems with mineral absorption can occur if concentrated fiber supplements are added to a plant-based diet already rich in fiber. Such supplements can be valuable for people eating low-fiber, animal-centered diets, but are both unnecessary and potentially damaging to those eating high-fiber, plant-based diets.

Fiber and Gas

Gas production is a normal, healthy function of the intestines. It is the result of bacteria in the large intestine using undigested carbohydrates (fiber) and releasing its by-products (hydrogen, carbon dioxide, methane, water, and short-chain fatty acids). This process appears to protect the colon against damage leading to cancer. It dilutes carcinogens, stimulates beneficial bacterial growth, favorably alters the acidity of the gut, and improves the function of the epithelial cells of the colon.

However, as wonderful as it may be for health, there comes a point after which it can cause significant physical and emotional trauma. Excessive gas production often creates bloating and painful cramping, unless of course you choose to pass the gas and risk the social consequences.

Fortunately, there are a number of steps you can take to reduce the discomfort and embarrassment involved with high fiber intakes. There are two distinct causes of gas production: fermentation of carbohydrates that reach the large intestine and swallowing of air. You can reduce the amount of air you swallow by eating more slowly, avoiding carbonated beverages and beer, not chewing gum or sucking on candy, and, if you wear dentures, making sure that they fit properly.

As for reducing the fermentation of carbohydrates, here are a few tips.

- Increase your intake of high-fiber foods gradually so your gastrointestinal system has time to adapt.

- Eat beans and other fibrous foods regularly. This will encourage the growth of bacteria that are more efficient at completely digesting bean sugars (thereby reducing gas production).

- Moderate your intake of foods that are particularly problematic, especially at first. Among the worst offenders are beans and vegetables of the cabbage family.

- Reduce the oligosaccharide (bean sugar) content of legumes before they are eaten. Always soak beans overnight and drain off the soaking water before cooking them. (Not soaking beans can increase gas by up to ten times.)

- Use more tofu and textured vegetable protein, which contain less of the problem sugars.

- Try lentils or other small legumes rather than larger beans, which seem to cause more problems.

■ Don't overeat. Overeating increases the amount of food that ends up undigested in the colon.

■ Take an enzyme to break down undigestible carbohydrates before they reach the colon.

■ Play detective. The main culprit for you could be something you don't suspect, such as mushrooms, onions, or celery.

■ Increase intake of noncarbonated beverages such as water or herbal teas.

PRACTICAL POINTER

Increase your fiber intake to 35 to 50 grams per day. The easiest and most beneficial way of accomplishing this is by eating a plant-based, whole foods diet, increase your fiber gradually and be sure to drink plenty of fluids when you do (6 to 8 glasses a day—preferably water and/or herbal tea.

Plant Protein

When most people think of protein, the first thing that comes to mind is meat—beef, pork, chicken, turkey, lamb, and fish. Next come eggs and dairy products like cheese, cottage cheese, and yogurt. For people with diabetes, the need for animal protein is reinforced by exchange lists that include a huge protein group called "meat and meat substitutes." It is little wonder that for many people the whole concept of plant protein seems rather foreign. It is time to tackle the myths and see plant protein for what it really is: another powerful ally in your fight for health.

Let's begin by considering the advantages of plant protein over animal protein.

■ Plants are high in fiber; meat, eggs, and dairy products are fiber-free.

■ Most plants are naturally low in fat (notable exceptions include nuts, seeds, and soy)—5 percent or less for most legumes. The fat they do contain is primarily unsaturated. Animal foods tend to be higher in fat, and the fat they contain is more highly saturated.

■ Plants are cholesterol-free; meat is high in cholesterol. Plants also contain phytosterols that help reduce cholesterol absorption.

■ The protein in plants lowers blood cholesterol levels; the protein in animal foods raises blood cholesterol levels.

■ Plants come conveniently packaged with many protective phytochemicals; animal foods contain no phytochemicals.

■ Plants provide calcium; meat is very low in calcium and increases calcium losses in the urine.

■ High protein intakes from meat can compromise kidney function, while plant protein appears to be protective.

Even after having digested all of that, you may still have the gut feeling that some animal protein is necessary for health. There are two questions that seem to concern people about protein.

1. Can I Get Enough Protein from Plants?

There is no question that we need sufficient protein. It is essential for building body tissues like bones, muscles, blood cells, digestive enzymes, and antioxidant enzymes. As you recall, people with diabetes may need a little extra protein, about 1 gram of protein per kg of body weight (just under a half gram of protein per pound body weight). For most people, protein needs are in the range of 60 to 90 grams a day, depending on body size. (See table 3.8 for a sample plant-based diet providing 90 grams of protein.) Referring back to table 3.6, you can see it would not be difficult to achieve these amounts on a plant-based diet.

Another way to look at protein needs is the percent of calories that should come from protein. About 15 percent of calories from protein is generally recommended. Beans are the protein powerhouses of the plant kingdom, providing about 20 to 30 percent of their calories from protein,

TABLE 3.8   Grams of Protein from Plants (1,800 calorie diet)

Breakfast	Lunch	Dinner	Snacks
Whole grain cereal with 1 Tbsp. walnuts and dried cranberries, 1 cup	Bean soup, 1 cup	BBQ tofu, 4 oz.	Raw vegetables, 2 cups
	Green salad with 1 Tbsp. pumpkin seeds, 3 cups	Broccoli/red pepper stir-fry, 1 cup	Grapefruit, 1
Soymilk, 1 cup	Flax dressing, 1 Tbsp.	Baked potato, 1 small	Rye crisp bread, 2
Blueberries, ½ cup		Banana-maple/walnut	Vegetarian deli slices, 2
	Cherries, 1 cup	"ice cream," 1 cup	
17 grams protein	**21 grams protein**	**34 grams protein**	**18 grams protein**

with soybeans, tofu, and veggie "meats" all being significantly higher. Vegetables provide about 15 to 40 percent of calories from protein, with a few exceptions, including root vegetables, which contain only about 7 to 12 percent of calories from protein. Grains, nuts, and seeds range from about 7 to 17 percent protein, with rice being on the low end. Fruits are generally lower in protein with about 1 to 10 percent of calories as protein.

By eating a variety of plant foods, it is not difficult to meet recommended intakes for protein. However, if you are on a calorie-reduced diet, as are many people with type 2 diabetes, you may have to pay a little closer attention to protein than you would otherwise. Some of the things you can do to increase your plant protein intake are

■ Eat legumes and products made from legumes such as tofu, tempeh, and soynuts on a daily basis.

■ Include some low-fat veggie "meats," which are especially concentrated protein foods.

■ Use a higher-protein nondairy milk such as soymilk, rather than rice milk or almond milk.

■ Add soy protein powder to shakes, muffins, and other prepared foods.

■ Select higher-protein grains, nuts, and seeds, such as quinoa, amaranth, almonds, peanuts, and pumpkin seeds.

2. Isn't the Quality of Plant Protein Inferior to Animal Protein?

Most people firmly believe that animal protein is necessary for human health and that plant protein is not only inferior, but actually lacking in essential amino acids and therefore inadequate to support growth and tissue repair. Animal foods are thought to be the primary source of all essential amino acids. But in truth, plants are the primary source of all essential amino acids. The reason that they are "essential" is because animals, including humans, can't make them. All animals get their essential amino acids, directly or indirectly, from plants (directly by eating plants or indirectly by eating other animals that ate plants). It makes no sense that we can't get sufficient protein from plants, when they are the original source of all essential amino acids.*

---

*Amino acids are the building blocks of protein. There are twenty-two amino acids, nine of which humans cannot make and must obtain from the diet. These nine amino acids are called essential amino acids. Once in our tissues, the essential amino acids from plant and animal foods are virtually identical.

Mono and Polyunsaturated Fat

Let's face it; fat gets a lot of bad press. We blame all sorts of health problems on fat—and with good reason. As you know, excessive amounts of saturated fats and trans fatty acids contribute to disease. It is little wonder some people end up becoming fat phobic, shunning not only visible fat like margarine and oil, but products with added fat and foods that are naturally high in fat. The flaw in this logic is that not all fat is damaging to health. In fact, some types of fat are quite harmless, and still others are essential to life. That's right—we need fat. It provides energy, supplies insulation, protects vital organs, provides physical padding, and is necessary for the absorption of many vitamins, minerals, and phytochemicals. Specific types of fat are also required for the formation of healthy cell membranes and the maintenance of cell integrity, permeability, shape, and flexibility. They are critical to the development and functioning of the brain and nervous system, and are involved in the production of hormonelike substances called eicosanoids, which regulate many organ systems. These special fats are known as essential fatty acids (EFAs) because our very survival depends on them.

Monounsaturated fats have been shown to have beneficial effects on health, protecting against chronic diseases. They are neutral or slightly beneficial in their effects on total cholesterol and do not decrease HDL ("good cholesterol")—in fact, they may even slightly increase it. There is some evidence that monounsaturated fats reduce blood pressure and enhance blood flow. For people with diabetes, monounsaturated fats have been shown to improve blood sugar control without the increase in triglyceride levels that often occurs with diets high in refined carbohydrates. The main dietary sources of monounsaturated fats are olives, olive oil, canola oil, avocados, most nuts (except for walnuts and butternuts), high-oleic sunflower oil, and high-oleic safflower oil.

Polyunsaturated fats are extremely important because it is within this group that the essential fatty acids reside. There are two distinct families of polyunsaturated fats, each with unique properties and effects. They are known as the omega-6 family and the omega-3 family, and both are vital to health. Some of these substances may be new to you, but you will probably be hearing about them more and more in the news. Details about each of these families of polyunsaturated fats are provided in table 3.9.

Almost all North American diets provide plenty of omega-6 fatty acids (and in some cases, possibly even too much), but insufficient omega-3 fatty acids.

TABLE 3.9   Omega-6 and Omega-3 Fatty Acid Families

	Omega-6 Fatty Acid Family	Omega-3 Fatty Acid Family
Essential Fatty Acid (EFA) —fatty acid we must get from food; we cannot make in our bodies	Linoleic acid (LA)	Alpha-linolenic acid (ALA)
Food Sources of EFAs	Sunflower, safflower, corn, soy, grapeseed, sesame, cottonseed, and hempseed oils, grains, seeds (except flaxseeds), walnuts, butternuts, soybeans, wheat germ.	Flaxseed and flaxseed oil, hempseed and hempseed oil, canola oil, walnuts and walnut oil, soybeans, soy products and soy oil, greens, some seaweed.
Highly Unsaturated Fatty Acids (HUFA) —fats we make from EFAs or obtained directly from food	Gamma-linolenic acid (GLA) Arachidonic acid (AA)— AA is efficiently produced from linoleic acid (LA) in the body	Eicosapentaenoic acid (EPA) Docosahexaenoic acid (DHA)—Conversion from alpha-linolenic acid (ALA) is very low (0% to 10 %), thus a direct source may be advised.
Sources of HUFA	GLA—borage, black current, primrose and hempseed oil, spirulina. AA—meat, poultry, dairy products.	EPA—fish, especially cold-water fish, some seaweeds. DHA—fish, especially cold-water fish, eggs (omega-3-rich eggs are highest), DHA-rich microalgae.
Health Effects for People with Type 2 Diabetes	GLA improves nerve function and prevents nerve deterioration. Too much AA can have negative consequences for heart health, increasing blood pressure, blood clotting, and inflammation.	EPA and DHA improve the fluidity of cell membranes, increasing their sensitivity to insulin. Omega-3 fatty acids protect heart health by reducing blood pressure, blood clotting, inflammation, and cardiac arrhythmias.

	Omega-6 Fatty Acid Family	Omega-3 Fatty Acid Family
Amount—How much of these fatty acids do I need?	About 5-8% of calories or 6-9 grams per 1,000 calories.	About 2% of calories or about 2.2 grams per 1,000 calories.
Concerns	Too much omega-6 fatty acid can reduce our ability to make the long-chain omega-3 fatty acids, EPA and DHA. This is especially important for those not eating EPA and DHA directly.	People with diabetes may have a reduced ability to make EPA and DHA compared to the general population. Some experts suggest that a direct source of these fatty acids be used.

Getting Enough Essential Fatty Acids in the Diet

It is extremely important to ensure sufficient essential fatty acids in the diet. For most people that means increasing intake of omega-3 fatty acids and keeping omega-6 fatty acids about the same, or in some cases reducing them. There is reasonable evidence to suggest that people with diabetes may benefit from direct sources of the long-chain fatty acids GLA, EPA, and DHA (which are more highly unsaturated), rather than relying on their bodies to make them from essential fatty acids (LA and ALA).

1. Include adequate sources of alpha-linolenic acid (omega-3) in the diet. Your best sources are flaxseeds, flaxseed oil, hempseeds, hempseed oil, canola oil, walnuts, and green leafy vegetables. Most people need about 3 to 5 grams of alpha-linolenic acid (ALA) each day. Flaxseeds are by far the richest source of ALA in the diet (57 percent of the fat is ALA). One teaspoon (5 mL) of flaxseed oil, plus your usual intake of vegetables, walnuts, and other foods provides ample ALA. (See table 3.10 for the alpha-linolenic acid content of selected foods.)

2. Consider including sources of EPA and/or DHA in your diet. The richest source of EPA and DHA is cold-water fish. High-fat, cold-water fish contains up to 1,600 mg DHA and 1,000 mg EPA per 3.5 oz. (100 gram) serving. EPA is also found in seaweed, with up to 30 percent of the fat in some varieties being EPA. (Seaweed has little DHA.) However, seaweed is so low in fat that you'd need to eat a lot of it to make a significant contribution to your intake. One hefty serving of 100 grams of seaweed provides about 100 mg of EPA.

DHA is also found in microalgae (microscopic sea plants), some of which contain as much as 40 percent DHA by dry weight. While we don't eat microalgae, it is currently being cultivated, extracted, and sold as a DHA supplement with 100 to 300 mg DHA per capsule. Eggs from chickens fed flax or DHA-rich microalgae are also reasonable DHA sources, providing 60 to 150 mg DHA per egg. For those wishing to supplement, 1,000 mg of DHA and EPA from fish oil, or 200 to 300 mg of DHA from microalgae is recommended.

3. Consider including a direct source of GLA in your diet. Very few foods contain GLA. Hempseed oil and spirulina contain small amounts. If you wish to supplement with GLA, about 250 mg per day is generally suggested for people with diabetes. This could be obtained from 1 gram of borage oil, 1.5 grams of black current oil, or 2.5 grams of primrose oil.

4. Select foods and oils rich in monounsaturated fat. By choosing foods and oils with monounsaturated fats, we avoid getting too much omega-6 fatty acids. If you use concentrated fats and oils, choose olive oil, canola oil, high-oleic (high monounsaturated) sunflower or safflower oil, and nut oils. Extra-virgin olive oil is generally the only unrefined oil available on supermarket shelves, so it's an excellent choice. If you choose canola oil, opt for organic. (About 70 percent of the canola oil in supermarkets is made from genetically engineered crops.) Whole foods rich in monounsaturated fats are your best

TABLE 3.10 Omega-3 (ALA) Content of Selected Foods

FOOD	OMEGA-3 FATTY ACIDS (ALA) GRAMS
Flaxseed oil, 1 Tbsp. (15 mL)	8.0
Hempseed oil, 1 Tbsp. (15 mL)	2.7
Walnuts, 1 oz. (28 g)	2.7
Flaxseeds, 1 Tbsp. (15 mL)	2.6
Canola oil, 1 Tbsp. (15 mL)	1.6
Soybeans, 1 cup (250 mL) cooked	1.1
Soybean oil, 1 Tbsp. (15 mL)	1.0
Leafy greens, 1 cup (250 mL) raw	0.1
Wheat germ, 2 Tbsp. (30 mL)	0.1

sources of these fats—nuts, olives, and avocados. Use them in moderation because they are loaded with calories!

5. Enjoy omega-6-rich foods, but limit oils rich in omega-6 fatty acids. Food such as sunflower seeds, pumpkin seeds, tofu, and wheat germ are great sources of omega-6 fatty acids and a healthful addition to your diet. However, it is best to limit your use of oils rich in omega-6 fatty acids because they can cause omega-6 intakes to climb too high.

6. Avoid excessive saturated fat and trans fatty acids

Should People with Type 2 Diabetes Eat Fish?

There is no doubt that fish is the most concentrated, most economical source of long-chain omega-3 fatty acids. The unique essential fatty acid content combined with its relatively low saturated fat content gives fish a rather distinct nutritional advantage over red meat and poultry. However, fish is far from being a knight in shining armor, and there are plenty of sound reasons to abstain. For starters, fish often comes from polluted waters containing high levels of heavy metals such as mercury, lead, and cadmium, and industrial pollutants such as PCBs, DDT, and dioxin. You also run the risk of being one of the hundreds, perhaps thousands, of people in North America who contract a food-borne illness from eating fish each day.

There are also compelling ecological and ethical arguments against fish consumption. The Natural Resources Defense Council (NRDC) estimates that about 70 percent of the world's fish populations are now fully fished, overexploited, depleted, or slowly recovering. A recent report out of Dalhouse University warns that we have only 10 percent of all large fish left in the sea. The report reveals that industrial fisheries take only 10 to 15 years to reduce any given fish population to 10 percent of its original size.

If you decide to forgo fish, you can be assured that you can get sufficient omega-3 fatty acids without it. Include good sources of alpha-linolenic acid in your diet, and consider taking a microalgae-based DHA supplement. While microalgae supplements don't provide any EPA, about 10 percent of the DHA we consume is converted back to EPA.

PRACTICAL POINTER

Do include some fat in your diet. Most of your fat should come from whole plant foods like nuts, seeds, avocados, olives, and soy. If you use concentrated oils, select those that are mainly monounsaturated, like extra-virgin olive oil or organic canola oil. Be sure to include omega-3-rich foods in your daily diet.

NUTRITION GUIDELINES FOR PEOPLE WITH TYPE 2 DIABETES

■ Reduce your intake of saturated fats to not more than 7 percent of total calories (primary sources: meat, poultry, dairy products, eggs, and tropical oils).

■ Keep trans fatty acids below 1 percent of calories (primary sources: processed foods containing hydrogenated or partially hydrogenated fats).

■ Limit your cholesterol intake to not more than 300 mg a day, and 200 mg a day for those with LDL cholesterol levels greater than 100 mg/dL (2.6 mmol/L) (primary sources: animal foods—meat, dairy products, and eggs).

■ Minimize your use of refined carbohydrates (simple sugars and starches in processed foods).

■ Keep sodium intake under 2,400 mg (6 grams or 1 teaspoon salt) per day (primary sources: processed foods, condiments, table salt).

■ If you use alcohol, limit intake to not more than one drink a day for women and two drinks a day for men.

■ Drink at least six to eight cups of water each day.

■ Ensure sufficient, but not excessive, protein intake. Get most of your protein from plant foods.

■ Select organic foods when you have a choice.

■ Base your diet on a variety of colorful, whole plant foods.

■ Eat at least seven to ten servings of vegetables and fruits each day.

■ Eat at least five servings of whole grains each day.

■ Include at least one serving of legumes in your daily diet.

■ Eat small portions of nuts and seeds daily.

■ Include sufficient servings of fiber-rich foods to provide 35 to 50 grams of fiber each day.

■ Include reliable sources of essential fatty acids and long-chain fatty acids GLA, EPA, and DHA in your daily diet.

CHAPTER 4

Healthy Weight For Life

W elcome to the land of "over" plenty, where the bulk of the population is dangerously overfed and overweight. In fact, overconsumption is now considered an epidemic in North America and the fastest growing form of malnutrition in the world. According to the State of the World 2000 report, the number of people suffering from overconsumption hit 1.2 billion—roughly the same as the number of people suffering the more commonly recognized form of malnutrition—hunger. People of all ages are getting fatter, and at alarming rates. The proportion of U.S. adults over twenty-five years old who are overweight soared from 25 percent in 1950 to 61 percent in 2002. Along with the increased girth comes an escalation in chronic diseases like type 2 diabetes. Over the past thirty years, the incidence of type 2 diabetes has tripled.

Even more frightening is the age of people who are developing the disease. At one time type 2 diabetes was called "adult-onset diabetes" because it generally affected individuals over fifty years of age. Over the past decade, increases in the rates of type 2 diabetes in younger people have been stunning. Between 1990 and 1998 rates climbed 70 percent in 30- to 39-year-olds, and 40 percent in 40- to 49-year-olds. Most alarming is the rise in type 2 diabetes in children and adolescents. In the past, over 95 percent of the diabetes in children was type 1, insulin-dependent diabetes, related to an infection or allergy-triggered loss of insulin production. Today, an estimated one-third of all newly diagnosed diabetes in children and teens in America is type 2.

IS BEING OVERWEIGHT SUCH A BIG DEAL?

Unfortunately, it is. You are well aware that obesity increases your risk of type 2 diabetes, but it also elevates your risk of most of the other chronic degenerative diseases plaguing the Western world. The strength of this link is so powerful it cannot be ignored. Among the most concerning consequences are

Heart disease and stroke—Being overweight contributes to high blood pressure, high cholesterol, high triglycerides, and angina (chest pain), and can markedly increase your chances of sudden heart attack or stroke.

Cancer—Overweight women suffer more breast, uterine, cervical, ovarian, gallbladder, and colon cancers, while overweight men are at an elevated risk for cancers of the colon, rectum, and prostate.

Osteoarthritis—Excess body weight increases the risk of osteoarthritis, probably by placing extra pressure on our joints and eroding the cartilage tissue that cushions the joints and provides protection.

Sleep apnea—Sleep apnea causes pauses in breathing during sleep, often marked by heavy snoring and snorting breaths following sometimes fairly prolonged lapses in breathing. In some cases severe daytime sleepiness (narcolepsy), hypertension, or even heart failure have developed due to this abnormality of breath control. (See page 155 for more information). Risk for sleep apnea is significantly higher in overweight individuals.

Gout—Gout is the product of high levels of uric acid in the blood. It causes painful swelling in the joints, usually affecting one joint at a time. The most common site affected is the big toe, but it is also seen in the ankle, knee, elbow, wrist, and finger joints. Overweight people are at greater risk for gout, and the risk increases progressively with higher body weights.

Gallbladder disease—Being overweight significantly increases risk of both gallbladder disease and gallstones. Rapid, significant weight loss can actually increase your chances of developing gallstones. Gradual weight loss of about one to two pounds a week is less likely to trigger attacks.

To make matters worse, a recent report found that obesity is contributing significantly more to America's rising health care and drug costs than smoking and alcohol abuse. Even more stunning, the report suggests that being obese effectively ages you twenty years. That puts an obese thirty-year-old in the same risk group as a normal-weight fifty-year-old for developing serious medical problems like cancer, heart disease, and diabetes.

There is no doubt that there are many overweight people who live a healthy lifestyle, including regular exercise and a nutritious diet—although they *are* taking in more than they burn off! These individuals are definitely at a reduced risk of complications when compared to those overweight individuals who are sedentary and eat an unhealthful diet. This is one of the reasons it is so important to keep health as your focus. Even small changes can add up to big rewards, wherever you are on the continuum of body size or weight.

How Do I Determine My Healthy Body Weight?

The most accurate way of assessing whether or not you are overweight or obese is to calculate how much of your body weight is fat. A body fat level greater than 17 percent in men and 27 percent in women indicates overweight, while a body fat level of greater than 25 percent in men and 31 percent in women indicates obesity. Unfortunately, getting accurate body fat measurements can be difficult and costly. Thus, a simple tool called *body mass index (BMI)* is commonly used for estimating total body "fatness." It is recommended for people between the ages of twenty and sixty-five years and is not considered valid for children, pregnant or nursing women, or for individuals with very large muscle mass, such as weight lifters or bodybuilders. After age sixty-five, body fat naturally increases, and higher BMIs are not as closely associated with disease in this age group. The greater your BMI is above 25, the more you are overweight and the more likely you are to develop health problems as a result. To find your BMI, plot your height and weight on table 4.1.

TABLE 4.1 — Body Mass Index (BMI)

HEIGHT IN INCHES

WT/LBS	60	61	62	63	64	65	66	67	68	69	70	71	72	73	74	75	76
100	20	19	18	18	17	17	16	16	15	15	14	14	14	13	13	12	12
105	21	20	19	19	18	17	17	16	16	16	15	15	14	14	13	13	13
110	21	21	20	19	19	18	18	17	17	16	16	15	15	15	14	14	13
115	22	22	21	20	20	19	19	18	17	17	17	16	16	15	15	14	14
120	23	23	22	21	21	20	19	19	18	18	17	17	16	16	15	15	15
125	24	24	23	22	21	21	20	20	19	18	18	17	17	16	16	16	15
130	25	25	24	23	22	22	21	20	20	19	19	18	18	17	17	16	16
135	26	26	25	24	23	22	22	21	21	20	19	19	18	18	17	17	16
140	27	26	26	25	24	23	23	22	21	21	20	20	19	18	18	17	17
145	28	27	27	26	25	24	23	23	22	21	21	20	20	19	19	18	18
150	29	28	27	27	26	25	24	23	23	22	22	21	20	20	19	19	18
155	30	29	28	27	27	26	25	24	24	23	22	22	21	20	20	19	19
160	31	30	29	28	27	27	26	25	24	24	23	22	22	21	21	20	19
165	32	31	30	29	28	27	27	26	25	24	24	23	22	22	21	21	20
170	33	32	31	30	29	28	27	27	26	25	24	24	23	22	22	21	21
175	34	33	32	31	30	29	28	27	27	26	25	24	24	23	22	22	21
180	35	34	33	32	31	30	29	28	27	27	26	25	24	24	23	22	22
185	36	35	34	33	32	31	30	29	28	27	27	26	25	24	24	23	23
190	37	36	35	34	33	32	31	30	29	28	27	26	26	25	24	24	23
195	38	37	36	35	34	33	32	31	30	29	28	28	27	26	25	24	24
200	39	38	37	35	34	33	32	31	30	30	29	28	27	26	26	25	24
205	40	39	37	36	35	34	33	32	31	30	29	29	28	27	26	26	25
210	41	40	38	37	36	35	34	33	32	31	30	29	28	28	27	26	26
215	42	41	39	38	37	36	35	34	33	32	31	30	29	28	28	27	26
220	43	42	40	39	38	37	36	35	34	33	32	31	30	29	28	27	27
225	44	43	41	40	39	37	36	35	34	33	32	31	31	30	29	28	27
230	45	43	42	41	39	38	37	36	35	34	33	32	31	30	30	29	28
235	46	44	43	42	40	39	38	37	36	35	34	33	32	31	31	29	29
240	47	45	44	43	41	40	39	38	36	35	34	33	33	31	31	30	29
245	48	46	45	43	42	41	40	39	37	36	35	34	33	32	32	30	30
250	49	47	46	44	43	42	40	39	38	37	36	35	34	33	32	31	30

BMI less than 19: may indicate underweight

BMI 19–24.9: healthful weight for most people

BMI 25–29.9: indicates overweight

BMI more than 30: indicates obesity

Note: Overweight is also defined as 10% above healthy weight and obesity as 20% above healthy weight.

BMI has limited value for some people. For example, it does not factor in muscle mass, so very muscular people will have a high BMI, but low body fat. In addition, very short people (less than 5 feet) may have higher BMIs than would be expected relative to their size. There is also far greater variability in healthful body weights than what we once thought. A person may be significantly larger than current ideals and still be at a very healthful weight for their build.

People with a BMI of 30 or greater have a fivefold greater risk of diabetes than people with a BMI of 25 or less. Indeed, one large study of a group of women between thirty and fifty-five years looked at type 2 diabetes risk relative to body weight. Risk for diabetes in these women, based on their BMI, was compared to those with a BMI of less than 22. The results were astonishing (see table 4.2 below).

TABLE 4.2	BMI Increase in Risk of Type 2 Diabetes

Risk of type 2 diabetes in women relative to those with BMIs of less than 22

BMI	RISK
25-26.9	8.1 times higher
27-28.9	5.8 times higher
29-30.9	27.6 times higher
31-32.9	40.3 times higher
33-34.9	54.0 times higher
35+	93.2 times higher

from Colditz, G. A., et al.

In addition to weight, the distribution of body fat plays an important role in predicting your risk of diabetes. People who accumulate fat in the abdomen and in the upper part of their body (apple-shaped) are at greater risk for diabetes than those who collect fat in their legs, hips, and buttocks (pear-shaped). The best way to determine body shape is to measure your waist. A waist circumference of greater than 35 inches in women and 40 inches in men is associated with an increased risk of diabetes. If you are overweight and carry much of your weight around the abdominal area, your risk can be further determined depending on whether or not the fat is accumulated in and around body organs (visceral fat) or just under the skin (subcutaneous fat). Those with greater levels of visceral fat are at higher risk for diabetes, poor glycemic control, and heart disease than those with mostly subcutaneous fat.

Why are so many of us overweight or obese?

Why wouldn't we be? We've created an ideal environment for weight gain. Almost every aspect of our society supports overeating and underactivity. We no longer spend hours running through dense forests in search of food. We simply open the refrigerator or freezer, pop a ready-made snack or meal into the microwave, and presto, instant satisfaction. If we get a little hankering for something when we are in the car, we don't have to take a step outside. We just slip into a drive-through fast-food restaurant and load up on whatever our heart desires. If we happen to be in the mall, treats beckon us at every turn. At work, there is often the lure of a cafeteria or at the very least a few vending machines. We are surrounded by an abundance of food and, not surprisingly, it shows.

The icing on the cake is a parallel decline in physical activity, the polar opposite of what the situation calls for. Few of us ever experience the hard physical labor of our forefathers. Today, most people have sedentary jobs, many of which involve sitting at a desk for much, if not all, of the day. In our spare time we watch television, play video games, or surf the Net. Every convenience possible has been developed to help reduce energy expenditure —remote controls, bread machines, electric can openers, elevators, electric mixers, dishwashers, and the list goes on. The problem is that the human body was built to endure famine, to get the most out of each calorie. People with type 2 diabetes tend to be particularly blessed with metabolic efficiency. It may feel like a curse, given our current level of affluence, but it was meant to provide a distinct survival advantage in the face of adversity.

While too much food and too little exercise are technically the cause of overweight, this is rarely the whole story. For many people, overweight has as much to do with emotions, self-preservation, and social pressure as it does with overeating and underactivity. Many people eat to satisfy an emotional hunger for companionship, joy, passion, or love rather than to satisfy true physical hunger. This is often referred to as "emotional eating" and is well recognized as a major contributor to overweight. Others use food as a means of constructing walls around themselves that protect against intimacy and pain. Food never judges, never condemns, and always comforts. These apparent advantages are deceiving, as they come at an enormous cost to both physical and emotional well-being. The struggle with weight is often made worse by the society's constant pressure to be thin. The reaction to this pressure is often years of yo-yo dieting, sending our bodies into conservation mode, making them even more efficient metabolic machines, jealously guarding every fat store and every calorie taken in for the next time of famine.

Overweight is caused by a complex interplay of many factors, unique to each individual. As you might expect, there are as many proposed solutions as there are causes, which collectively make up the amazing multi-billion-dollar weight loss industry.

THE WEIGHT LOSS INDUSTRY— PROMISES, PROMISES, PROMISES

Melt pounds overnight! Eat all you want and lose weight! Lose thirty pounds in a month without dieting! It is awfully tempting to buy into every weight loss promise that comes along. However, if a safe and simple cure for obesity really existed, would 61 percent of the population over twenty-five years of age be overweight? The sad reality is that upwards of 95 percent of weight loss efforts fail. So, if you set out in search of a weight loss wonder, make sure you do so with eyes wide open.

Diets for Every Season

How many diets have you tried? How many have succeeded? Weight loss diets are generally designed to produce a calorie deficit or to ensure you take in fewer calories than you burn, so you'll lose weight. Most succeed in this task. When it comes to weight loss, whether you eat grapefruit, cabbage soup, or bacon and eggs matters far less than the number of calories you consume. The obvious question is, if most diets succeed in producing weight loss, what's the problem? It's really very simple; they end. When they do, the weight creeps back on. Unfortunately, in many cases the diet sends your metabolism on a downward swing, and your body becomes even more efficient than it was before. This means that in addition to gaining back the lost weight, you may end up with a bonus of a few extra pounds. There is one sure way of determining if a diet has any hope of success in the long term. Ask yourself this question: *Can I eat this way for the rest of my life?*

If the answer is no, it's a waste of time and effort—unless of course you want to lose weight just long enough to fit into a certain outfit for some special occasion! The only way a diet will succeed permanently is if it becomes a way of life. In other words, there is no going back to the way you used to eat. For this reason, the diet must be nutritionally sound or your health will suffer.

Bearing in mind this vital question, let's consider the most popular weight loss diets of today.

One-Food or Few-Food Diets

Diets that are based on one or few foods get boring very quickly, and, as you might expect, are nutritionally inadequate. These diets are usually based on some "miracle food" like grapefruit, cabbage, or cottage cheese. The thought of eating this way for the rest of your life is absurd. For people with diabetes, these severely limited regimes are downright dangerous, especially for those on insulin. Diets that exclude many foods are less likely to provide a micronutrient-rich milieu in which a healthy metabolism can thrive. Variety may very well be "the spice of life," in that a spectrum of plant foods provides a safety net of protective phytonutrition, and any diet that would restrict that intake must be suspect.

Low-Carbohydrate, High-Protein Diets

The theory behind these diets is that cutting carbohydrates will result in reduced insulin response, less hunger, and less overeating. So it is not surprising that they are often promoted for people with insulin resistance and diabetes. The key problems with these regimens are they are often very high in fat, cholesterol, and animal protein, and very low in fiber, phytochemicals, and antioxidant nutrients. Some programs are far worse than others, with as much as 60 percent of calories from fat—much of it saturated fat! On weight loss diets, it is difficult to meet nutritional requirements when so many of the calories come from fat (which has very few nutrients). Some low-carbohydrate diets are more moderate in fat, with approximately 40 percent of calories from carbohydrates, 30 percent from protein, and the remaining 30 percent from fat. While vegetarian versions of these moderate programs can be safe and adequate, they need to be very carefully constructed to allow for sufficient fiber, phytochemicals, and antioxidants.

Very Low-Fat, High-Fiber Diets

As you may recall from chapter 2, very low-fat vegetarian diets can be effective choices for weight loss. However, to maximize their advantages, it is very important not to make refined carbohydrates a dietary staple, as this causes an increase in triglycerides and a decrease in "good" HDL cholesterol. Two major drawbacks of the very low-fat diets are that they may reduce the absorption of protective vitamins, minerals, and phytochemicals, and they may provide insufficient essential fatty acids. In addition, nutrient-dense, higher-fat plant foods such as nuts, seeds, avocados, and olives are often unnecessarily eliminated. These foods are important sources of trace minerals and the antioxidant vitamin E. So if you want to try a very low-fat diet, adjust fat up to a minimum of 15 percent of calories to allow for sufficient absorption of nutrients and phytochemicals, and adequate essential fatty acids.

Weight Watchers

This lifestyle program includes a comprehensive diet component. It is based on a points system, which monitors energy, fiber, and fat intakes. The diet is flexible, allowing for both vegetarian and vegan options. It is also nutritionally sound, and safe for people with type 2 diabetes. The main pitfall is the tedious task of calculating points for each food consumed. While most people are not willing to count points forever, in many cases it serves to educate participants about the nutritional content of foods, thereby helping to build more healthful habits. For those interested in group support, Weight Watchers is a great choice.

Weight Loss Clinics

There are several weight control clinics that offer a host of special food products to aid in weight loss. While these programs can be very effective in the short term, few people will stay on packaged foods indefinitely. While such programs can offer excellent personal support, they are expensive and impractical in the long term.

THE BOTTOM LINE

Don't get caught up in claims of diet miracles. There are no miracle foods and no quick fixes. The real key to finding a diet that will help you achieve a healthy body weight for life is to find one that promotes permanent, positive changes in eating habits.

PILLS AND POTIONS...MAGIC BULLETS?

T he promise of popping a pill each day or drinking a special herbal tea and watching fat melt away is universally appealing to dieters. It comes as no surprise that those who seek a solution, with wallet in hand, will have a few thousand options to choose from. Some offer reasonable support, some are totally useless, and still others are risky.

Prescription Drugs

Swallowing a pill seems so much easier than changing your entire way of life. If only it were that simple! Prescription medications for weight control are not everything most people hope for. The most common prescription medications used for weight loss are appetite suppressants. They work by reducing appetite or increasing feelings of fullness. Only a few years ago, when the most popular of these drugs were used in combination and sold as the popular weight loss aid fen-phen, a reported association with heart valve problems and primary pulmonary hypertension forced the withdrawal of the medications from the market. Common side effects of appetite suppressants include dry mouth, headaches, constipation, insomnia, palpitations, and slight increases in blood pressure. Most of these drugs are derivatives of "speed," or methamphetamine, which was the first of these popular medications to be released and widely used back in the 1950s, until its potential for serious addiction and organ damage became well appreciated.

One of the newest prescription drugs on the market is a fat blocker sold under the name Xenical (orlistat). It works by inhibiting enzymes responsible for fat breakdown, reducing fat absorption by about 30 percent. The side effects of Xenical are diarrhea, poor absorption of fat-soluble vitamins and phytochemicals, anal leakage, and urgency. Many people simply cannot tolerate the gastric lipase inhibition necessary to benefit from the Xenical program, and in truth, if you are unable to restrict your intake of fat, the very loose stool can become quite unbearable.

Another popular prescription weight loss medication is sibutramine, or Meridia. This drug helps control appetite by increasing the levels of certain hormones in the brain (mainly serotonin) which control appetite and hunger. It does appear to be relatively well tolerated in the short term, although side effects such as dry mouth, headache, constipation, and insomnia are not uncommon. There are all kinds of contraindications for using this drug. It can't be used by individuals on other drugs in the same class, including antidepressants such as Prozac and Paxil. It can't be used by people with blood pressure problems, because it increases blood pressure. It can be risky for those with heart disease, kidney disease, and liver disease. You get the picture.

THE BOTTOM LINE

Prescription medications are generally reserved for those with severe obesity problems (BMI over 30 for healthy individuals; over 27 for those with serious diseases), and come with risk of serious side effects and numerous contraindications. Most people using these medications quickly regain lost weight when the medication is stopped, thus if medications are used, it should only be in combination with diet and lifestyle programs. In dire circumstances, where self-control and routine nutritional approaches have been strongly attempted, medications may be justified.

Nonprescription Drugs, Herbs, and Teas

Medicinal herbs are largely unregulated, so quality, effectiveness, and safety can be highly variable. While some of these products may help kick start weight loss efforts, they are not necessary, nor are they ever the answer to long-term healthful weight. Here are some of the more common products you'll see on the market.

Metabolic Stimulants

Herbal fen-phen is an over-the-counter replacement for the once popular prescription medication. It is made from ephedra (ma huang) and a combination of other active ingredients such as St. John's wort, caffeine, and aspirin. Ephedra is on the FDA's list of dangerous diet supplements because of reports of adverse effects, including nervousness, headaches, tremors, insomnia, high blood pressure, irregular heart beat, chest pain, heart attack, stroke, seizures, and death. This is definitely one to steer clear of.

Several spices, including red pepper, ginger, mustard seed, cinnamon, and cardamom are also thought to boost metabolic rate. Kelp and other sea vegetables are said to increase metabolism by virtue of their iodine content and thyroid stimulation. While evidence is lacking, these herbs and seaweeds are relatively safe.

Appetite Suppressants

Phenylpropanolamine (PPA) is often found in appetite suppressants as well as cough and cold remedies. The FDA recently recommended that products containing PPA be removed from the market due to evidence linking it to increased risk of hemorrhagic (bleeding) stroke in women.

Chickweed is also used as an appetite suppressant. As far as appetite suppressants go, it is among the least harmful. *Garcinia cambogia* is another rising star in the weight loss world. It is used as both an appetite suppressant and a fat burner, and appears quite harmless.

Fat Blockers

The most popular "natural" fat blocker is chitosan, which is derived from chitin, a complex starch found in the exoskeleton of shellfish such as shrimp, lobster, and crabs. Like Xenical, it can reduce the absorption of fat-soluble vitamins and phytochemicals, very possibly doing more harm than good.

Laxatives

There are two main types of laxatives: bulking agents and stimulants. Both are commonly used in herbal weight loss formulas. Stimulants such as senna, cascara sagrada, and buckthorn work by irritating the system, often causing cramps and diarrhea. Bulking agents like ground flaxseed and psyllium, when consumed with sufficient water, increase feelings of fullness and help improve bowel function. They are gentler than stimulants and can be highly effective for those who struggle with getting sufficient fiber in their diet. Ground flaxseed is an especially good choice as it provides essential fatty acids, phytochemicals, and several trace minerals in addition to the fiber.

Combination Preparations

Among the most popular weight loss preparations on the market today are those that include several of the above mentioned active components. A popular combination includes an herbal laxative, an herbal diuretic, a stimulant herb like ma huang or ephedra, and an herb containing caffeine, such as guarana. These kinds of formulas should be approached with a great deal of skepticism, as the mix of several of these herbal medications along with physical exertion, and perhaps some dehydration resulting from excessive perspiration, have been linked to several deaths in teens at rave parties.

THE BOTTOM LINE

Don't rely on any supplement to provide an answer to your weight concerns. If you must experiment with supplements, stick to herbal appetite suppressants, spices, and psyllium or flaxseed (bulking agents) with lots of water. But remember, your best allies will always be whole foods, water, and exercise.

THE ROAD TO LIFELONG HEALTHY WEIGHT!

The ultimate goal is to fuel your body with foods that support health and healing. To do so you need to be able to recognize the difference between true physiological hunger and emotional hunger. When the distinction is clear, you can begin to fill various hungers in ways that nourish your spirit rather than feed your disease. Your food choices need to be a reflection of the powerful connection between those choices and your well-being, rather than a function of convenience or habit. A healthful lifestyle requires a balance of body, mind, and spirit; nourish each of them. Begin your transformation by thinking about what you want your life to be. Picture yourself there. Imagine being fit and healthy. Believe that you can achieve whatever you set your mind to. Recognize that every small step in the right direction goes a long way toward achieving your goals. These guidelines will help to keep your focus where it needs to be.

Seven Simple Steps to Lifelong Healthy Weight

1. Set Realistic Goals.

Think about your goals, both long- and short-term. Write them down. Be sure to include lots of minigoals you are confident that you can achieve. Don't expect to lose 30 pounds in a month. For permanent weight loss, aim for no more than one to two pounds a week. Appreciate every little bit of progress you make. Walking an extra five minutes a day, being content with a slightly smaller serving size, or watching a half hour less television—every positive change is worth celebrating.

Be sure not to fall into the trap of embarking on a diet that is ultralow in calories in hopes of producing big losses. When you cut caloric intake too severely, your metabolism slows down. You have to eliminate even more calories to continue losing weight—it becomes a downward spiral. It also becomes very difficult to meet nutrient needs. Most of all, such diets are not useful in the long term—remember you need to be able to eat this way permanently! It is far better to opt for a moderate energy intake while, at the same time, increasing energy expenditure with physical activity. For every 500 calorie per day deficit, you'll lose about a pound a week. So, the goal is to produce a deficit of 500 to 1,000 calories, which amounts to one to two pounds a week. You can accomplish this by using a combination of diet and exercise. For example, you can reduce energy intake by 500 calories and expend an extra 250 calories per day in physical activity. This will produce an average loss of 1½ pounds per week. For most women, 1,500 calories per day is a reasonable goal, while for most men, 1,800 calories per day would be about right.

Beware of weight scales, as they tell only one part of the story. Weight naturally fluctuates from day to day and from morning to night. With increased physical activity, muscle mass increases, and muscle weighs more than fat. Thus, while your weight may be unchanged, you are actually leaner. You can count on the way your clothes fit far more than what a scale reads! If you must weigh yourself, do so at the same time of the day, and make it no more than once a week.

2. Center your diet on whole plant foods.

Make vegetables, fruits, legumes, whole grains, and small amounts of nuts and seeds the foundation of your diet. Select a wide variety of fresh, whole foods processed without added fat, sugar, or salt. Minimize your use of refined and processed foods. This will help to maximize protective dietary components. It also ensures an adequate intake of dietary fiber, which increases food volume without adding calories. It also helps speed food through the digestive system, resulting in fewer calories being absorbed. In addition, fiber reduces hunger and improves satiety.

The following tips will help get you started:

- *Eat at least three to five servings of vegetables each day.* Leafy greens are especially important, so include at least one to two servings a day. Include as many low-carbohydrate vegetables as you like, but limit higher carbohydrate vegetables (i.e., potatoes, corn, and peas) to not more than three servings a day.

- *Eat two to four servings of fruits each day.* While fruit is low in fat, it does add calories to your diet and can increase triglycerides, so keep portions moderate. Go for whole fruit instead of juice. It is more filling and takes longer to eat. If you do drink fruit juice, squeeze the fruit yourself when you can.

■ *Include five to eight servings of grains per day.* Select mainly whole grains, and not more than two servings of refined grains each day. Whole grains are more slowly digested than refined grains, leaving you feeling satisfied for a longer time. When you eat whole grains, you tend to eat slightly less than when you eat refined grains. Your best choices are intact whole grains (i.e., millet, quinoa, barley, brown rice). Use these grains for puddings, hot breakfast cereal, pilafs, casseroles, soups, and salads.

■ *Include at least two to four servings of legumes (beans), and products made from legumes (tofu, tempeh, vegetable patties, etc.) in your diet each day.* They are our best sources of protein, as well as minerals such as iron and zinc. Legumes are also loaded with fiber, helping you to feel satisfied for a longer time. Experiment with all kinds of legumes. Sprout them, stew them, add them to salads and loaves, or just eat them as a side dish.

■ *Don't forget the nuts and seeds, but keep portions small.* Nuts and seeds are high in fat, providing about 175 to 225 calories per ¼-cup serving (16 to 20 grams of fat). Don't snack on them by the handful; rather, sprinkle them on a salad, or add a few to a loaf of bread or your breakfast cereal.

3. Use beverages to your advantage!

Beverages can wreak havoc with weight loss goals. A 12-ounce (375 mL) serving of lemonade, fruit punch, or soda pop can contain up to 150 calories. A typical milkshake chalks up 350 calories, as does a mere 8 ounces (250 mL) of nonalcoholic eggnog. Alcoholic beverages can also send your calories soaring. Twelve ounces (375 mL) of beer provides 110 to 170 calories, distilled spirits about 110 calories per 1½ ounces (45 mL), liqueurs 150 to 190 calories per 1½ ounces (45 mL), and wine about 80 calories per 4 ounces (125 mL). Even nutritious beverages like juice or soymilk can contribute up to 150 calories per 8 ounces (250 mL). So if you drink four or five calorie-rich beverages a day, you could take in an extra 500 to 1,000 calories.

While some beverages add nutritional value to the diet, you are generally better off eating whole foods, as they provide more fiber and greater satiety value. When you are cutting calories in an effort to lose weight, it makes little sense to waste them on nonnutritious beverages. Your very best bet for fluids is water. In addition to being calorie-free, water offers numerous benefits for health. One recent report, using data from the Adventist Health Study, found that people who consume five or more servings of water per day had remarkably reduced risk for fatal heart attacks or stroke (almost half that of those drinking only one to two glasses per day).

4. Limit fat intake to not more than 25 percent of calories

You may be wondering what 25 percent of calories amounts to in grams of fat, or how many grams it would be on a 15-percent-fat diet? Table 4.3 provides the answers. In the left-hand column you will see various levels of caloric intake. The next three columns provide the maximum number of grams of fat you can have within three levels of fat intake: 15, 20, and 25 percent.

Fat is two and a half times more concentrated in energy than carbohydrates or protein (100 calories per tablespoon [15 mL] versus 40 calories for carbohydrate or protein), so even modest portions of high-fat foods can be very energy dense. Your body also converts dietary fat to body fat very efficiently, using up only about 2.5 calories for every 100 calories of fat in the process. By contrast, it takes 20 or more calories to convert 100 protein or carbohydrate calories to body fat. If you want to minimize fat storage, it makes good sense to limit fat intake.

TABLE 4.3	Maximum Fat Grams in 15%, 20%, and 25% Fat Diets		
	Maximum Fat Grams (g)		
Caloric Intake	**15%**	**20%**	**25%**
1,200	20 g	27 g	33 g
1,400	23 g	31 g	37 g
1,600	27 g	36 g	44 g
1,800	30 g	40 g	50 g
2,000	33 g	44 g	55 g
2,200	37 g	50 g	62 g

While it is important to remember that some types of fat are far more damaging to health than others, all fats are created equal when it comes to calories. Whether it's pure lard or extra-virgin olive oil, fat provides almost 4,000 calories per pound. By contrast, a pound of cooked brown rice contains about 540 calories, a pound of apples about 250 calories, and a pound of lettuce about 65. It is interesting, however, to note that the type of fat consumed may affect hormone levels and metabolism. Polyunsaturated fats, especially omega-3 fatty acids, appear to increase metabolic rates relative to saturated fats.

To reduce total fat intake

■ Cut back on visible fats

   ✔ Limit use of oils, butter, and margarine. Try to keep your intake to one tablespoon or less per day.

   ✔ Avoid fried foods. Opt for baked, broiled, or steamed instead.

   ✔ Flavor foods with fresh lemon juice, wine, flavored vinegars, salsa, soy sauce, and a variety of herbs and spices instead of fat.

■ Reduce intake of hidden fats

   ✔ If you use dairy products, select nonfat alternatives or plant-based substitutes.

   ✔ If you use eggs, keep intake to four or less per week.

   ✔ Replace high-fat snack foods such as cookies, crackers, and granola bars with low-fat, whole grain alternatives. Be aware that many low-fat products simply replace the fat with sugar—this is no bargain for people with diabetes!

5. Build healthful habits.

Examine your habits and replace those that undermine your goals with better choices. Take one small step at a time. If you end up backsliding, don't consume yourself with guilt. Instead, work on ways to make your new healthful habits even more enjoyable. Begin this journey by following these helpful hints.

- Eat regular, moderately sized meals. Skipping meals can compromise your performance and leave you so hungry that you overeat at the next meal. People who eat breakfast burn more calories during the day and perform better than those who don't.

- Watch your portion sizes. The more food on your plate, the more you end up eating. Using a smaller plate can help minimize portion sizes.

- Eat slowly. This not only enables you to better appreciate your food, it can help reduce the amount you eat and improve digestion.

- Don't eat standing. Always put your food in a bowl or on a plate, and sit down to eat.

- Avoid eating while cooking. You may need to suck on a mint or chew a piece of gum if this is a major challenge for you.

- Keep your hands busy while watching TV to avoid snacking. Somehow, when you eat while watching TV, you seem to be less conscious of how much you consume. You may wish to do a craft, catch up on the ironing, or do some stretching exercises to keep yourself otherwise occupied.

- Pick nutritious foods when eating out. If you find yourself tempted while out, go for fresh fruit, fresh-squeezed juices, an Asian stir-fry, some popcorn, or a frozen yogurt. Steer clear of deep-fried foods and sweet baked goods.

6. Make physical activity a priority in your life.

Physical activity tends not to happen unless it becomes a real priority in your life. Exercise offers huge advantages when it comes to weight loss. It increases stamina, energy output, and metabolism. Here are a few tips to help get you started (see also chapter 8):

- Exercise daily. Your best choice for weight loss and overall health is moderate aerobic activity (such as brisk walking) combined with moderate resistance training (such as light weight training). Don't forget to stretch!
- Avoid labor-saving devices when you can. Take the stairs instead of the elevator, park a couple of blocks from work, and hide the remote control.
- Be adventurous. Join a hiking club, take tennis lessons, or go on a wilderness adventure.
- Don't avoid an activity because of your size. By being active, you are setting a great example for others and living life to its fullest.
- Aim for thirty to sixty minutes of exercise each day. If that is difficult for you to start with, try several short ten-minute bursts throughout your day.

7. Take care of your inner being.

It is so tempting to eat when there is food around or you're bored, tired, or stressed out. Learn to recognize real hunger and respect it. Don't eat if you aren't hungry, but don't deprive yourself if you are. If you're bored, go out somewhere. If you're tired, have a nap. If you're stressed out, walk with a friend, pray, or meditate. Pay attention to how foods affect your digestive system. Be mindful of these things when you make food selections.

Great health can be realized only when you take care of your inner being. It could mean facing struggles, both past and present, that are yet unresolved. It may also involve seeking out a support group or therapist who can help you deal with depression, abuse, or anger. Until these underlying issues are addressed, it will be much more difficult for you to realize your ultimate health goals and fully appreciate the person you are.

The next chapter will provide you with the tools you need to design a diet that really works for you.

CHAPTER 5

Designing the Diabetes Diet

T Now that you know what's hot and what's not in the world of nutrition, let's explore ways you can use this information to design a diet that really works for you. If you imagine a near-perfect day of food choices, what would it look like? What would you have for breakfast, lunch, dinner, and snacks? What would the food taste like? Would you be satisfied? If the idea of a diet makeover makes you break out in a cold sweat, you are not alone. Most people are creatures of habit and the very thought of change can be completely overwhelming. Relax; take a deep breath. This new, more healthful way of eating will not leave you feeling hungry or otherwise deprived. On the contrary, you will notice that high-fiber whole foods are very filling, allowing you to eat more, yet take in fewer calories. And, while many people imagine "healthy food" to be boring and rather unsavory, these foods can be even more enticing than your former favorites. Admittedly, like any other major lifestyle change, transforming your diet takes some time and commitment, but you will feel so much better that it will hardly seem like a sacrifice at all. Just think of it as the adventure of a lifetime, with unparalleled rewards.

There are wonderful support systems and well-qualified individuals who can help you construct a personal plan based on your unique needs and health goals. Begin by finding a registered dietitian who you feel comfortable working with. The American Dietetic Association has a website to assist you. In their pages called "Find a Dietitian," you can do a search for a dietitian in your area who has expertise in both diabetes and vegetarian diets. The website is: http://www.eatright.org/find.html. Dietitians of Canada offers a similar service at: http://www.dietitians.ca/find/i4.htm. Diabetes Educators (e.g., Certified Diabetes Educators [CDE] and the American Association of Diabetes Educators [AADE]) can also provide excellent support. These are health professionals (dietitians, physicians, registered nurses, occupational therapists, and others) with special skills and experience in assisting people with diabetes. Most communities also have support groups for people with diabetes. Contact your local branch of the American or Canadian Diabetes Association for information.

TOOLS OF THE TRADE: EXCHANGE LISTS AND CARBOHYDRATE COUNTING

You may have some personal experience with the tools that are commonly used to translate nutrition information into practical food choices for people with diabetes. The two most popular systems are exchange lists and carbohydrate counters.

Exchange systems, such as the Exchange Lists for Meal Planning (U.S.) and the Good Health Eating Guide (Canada), have evolved over several decades and offer a sensible, organized approach to meal planning for people with diabetes. In these systems, foods are grouped according to their carbohydrate, protein, and fat content. People are allotted a certain number of servings from each list at every meal and snack. They can choose the foods they prefer within each list, although guidelines for making nutritious selections generally accompany such systems. The U.S. Exchange Lists places foods in one of three groups: the carbohydrate group, the meat and meat substitutes group, and the fat group. The carbohydrate group includes five lists: starch (grains and starchy vegetables), fruit, milk, vegetables, and other carbohydrates. The meat and meat substitutes group includes four lists: very lean, lean, medium-fat, and high-fat. The fat group includes three lists: monounsaturated fat, polyunsaturated fat, and saturated fat. All "visible fats" and oils (fats and oils that you can see, such as vegetable oil, margarine, butter, and shortening, as well as fat on meat or poultry), in addition to a number of foods containing "hidden fats" such as nuts, seeds, avocados, olives, coconut, and sour cream, are included in the fat list. In the Canadian system, food choices are divided into seven groups: starch (including grains and starchy vegetables), fruit and vegetable, milk, protein, fat, sugar, and extras. Within most categories, there is a section highlighting foods that fit into more than one category. For example, potato chips are in the starch group, but they count and as one starch plus two fats; cheese is in the protein group, but counts as one protein plus one fat.

Carbohydrate counting is an approach to meal planning that focuses on the carbohydrate content of foods eaten. There are three levels of carbohydrate counting. In the first level, the person with diabetes and the dietitian determine the total amount of carbohydrates that will be eaten at each meal or snack. Once the goal is set, the person learns to determine the carbohydrate content of various portions of foods, using a carbohydrate counter reference book or exchange lists. In the second level, the person progresses to making adjustments in his or her medication, food, and activities based on measured blood sugar levels. This involves learning to identify blood sugar patterns, recognizing causes of blood sugar variations, and taking appropriate action to achieve desired blood sugars. The third, and most advanced, level of carbohydrate counting, involves using a person's carbohydrate-to-insulin ratio. This is determined using daily records of carbohydrates eaten. Use of ratios allows for considerable flexibility in food choices and portion sizes. This final level is used primarily by those using multiple insulin injections or an insulin pump.

These tools were designed to help achieve two primary goals: blood sugar control and healthful body weights. Both systems improve blood sugar control by ensuring an appropriate intake and distribution of carbohydrates throughout the day, which is especially important for people taking insulin or medications that stimulate insulin secretion. Carbohydrate counting may be the best choice where blood sugar control is concerned, as it allows for more precise matching of food and insulin. Both methods support weight management by controlling portion sizes and calories. Exchange systems may be more effective than carbohydrate counting in this regard because they monitor carbohydrate, protein, and fat intakes, while carbohydrate counting looks only at carbohydrate consumption. While these systems can be useful tools for people with diabetes, both, in our view, have limitations. Among the most significant drawbacks of these food tools are

1. *Neither system adequately distinguishes among different forms of carbohydrate.* With carbohydrate counting, the focus is the total carbohydrate content of foods. Of course, since animal foods and pure fats contain no carbohydrate, they may be erroneously viewed in a favorable light. In addition, the remarkably different effects of various forms of carbohydrate are not recognized, so that 50 grams of carbohydrate from white bread may be viewed as being equal to 50 grams of carbohydrates from beans. With the exchange systems, concerns are similar. The "starch" list includes everything from sugar-frosted cereal and fat-free potato chips to oatmeal and corn on the cob. The "other carbohydrates" list includes everything from hummus to white sugar. There is no clear indication that their health effects are remarkably different.

2. *Both systems favor animal over plant protein sources.* With carbohydrate counting, meat appears very favorable, as it contains zero carbohydrates, while plant protein sources are moderate or rich sources of carbohydrate. In the U.S. Exchange Lists, the value of plant protein foods seems highly underrated. Beans appear at the bottom of the very lean meat and substitutes list and are counted as a serving from two separate lists—one serving from the meat list and one serving from the starch list. There is no mention that their high fiber content provides important advantages over other foods in this group. Tofu, tempeh, and soymilk appear at the bottom of the medium-fat meat and substitutes list with no indication that they provide advantages in terms of protein, cholesterol, and saturated fat content. Peanut butter is included at the bottom of the high-fat meat and substitutes list, below pork and beef wieners, sausage, and bacon. All other nuts and seeds and their butters are excluded from the high-fat meat list, relegated instead to the "fat list." This makes little sense considering that many other nuts and seeds provide about the same amount of protein and fat as peanut butter. Furthermore, the exchange system does not acknowledge meat "alternatives" such as very low-fat veggie "meats," which are high in protein, low in fat, and cholesterol-free.

3. *Neither system fully recognizes the huge variations in health effects of different types of fat.* While the "fat" list separates sources of monounsaturated, saturated, and polyunsaturated fat, it includes healthful whole foods such as nuts, seeds, and their butters, avocados, and olives in the same category as pure fats. While these foods are rich in fat, they are highly protective due to

the quality of fat and the presence of phytochemicals and trace minerals; furthermore they provide some protein. When counted simply as "fat," they may be viewed as detrimental. Walnuts and seeds are included in the polyunsaturated group along with stick margarine. Placing these foods in the same category leads people to believe that they are nutritionally similar, when they are clearly worlds apart. Finally, there is no mention of rich sources of omega-3 fatty acids, which are especially important for people with diabetes.

THE PLANT-BASED, WHOLE-FOOD SOLUTION

The beauty of whole food, plant-based diets is that many of the problems inherent in these traditional tools of diabetes management are resolved with little effort at all. Each and every whole plant food contains unrefined carbohydrates and fiber. As a result, the vast majority of these foods have very respectable glycemic indexes. Thus, when you eat a variety of whole plant foods throughout the day, your carbohydrate intake will naturally be well distributed, providing that calories are held relatively constant. In addition, such diets generally provide about 35 to 50 grams of fiber, helping to satisfy your appetite without excessive calories. The quantity and quality of fat in such diets is also usually well within healthful limits when added concentrated fats and oils are used judiciously. Low-fat, plant-based diets have been shown to promote remarkable improvements in blood sugar control and weight loss in people with type 2 diabetes, even if the calories in the diets are not restricted.

Does that mean you can eat whatever whole plant foods you want, in whatever quantities you please? Well, not quite. You do need to consider portion sizes, fat content, and the nutritional value of the foods you select. For example, if you choose to eat a couple of avocados or a cup of nuts each day, you'll have a difficult time keeping calories within a range that would promote weight loss. The key to health is to include a wide variety of plant foods, ensuring a balance of essential nutrients. If you are eating a completely plant-based diet, you also need to think about what we call "nutrients of concern"—primarily vitamins B_{12} and D, calcium, and omega-3 fatty acids. These are nutrients that may be low, even when an excellent variety of whole foods is provided. (See table 5.8 on pages 119-20 for a discussion of these nutrients.) For many people, having a tool to help determine food choices and portion sizes can be helpful, especially in the early stages of the transition to a plant-based diet. For this reason, we have developed a "Plant-Based Food Guide for People with Diabetes." (See figure 5.1.) This guide can provide you

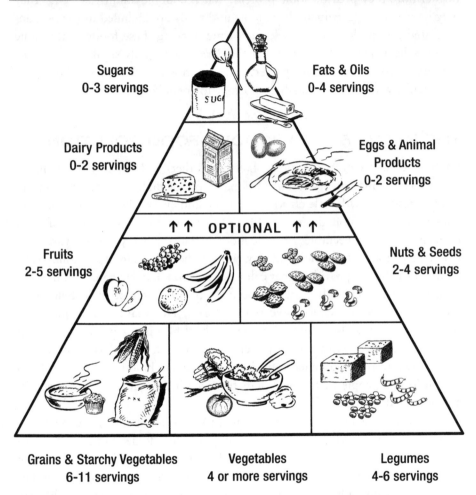

FIGURE 5.1 — Plant-Based Food Guide For People with Diabetes

Sugars
0-3 servings

Fats & Oils
0-4 servings

Dairy Products
0-2 servings

Eggs & Animal Products
0-2 servings

↑ ↑ OPTIONAL ↑ ↑

Fruits
2-5 servings

Nuts & Seeds
2-4 servings

Grains & Starchy Vegetables
6-11 servings

Vegetables
4 or more servings

Legumes
4-6 servings

with direction as you shift towards a plant-based diet, or it can be used as a plant-based "exchange system." It will also help you ensure that all your nutrient needs are met. Following the guide will provide a diet of approximately 55 to 65 percent carbohydrates, 20 to 25 percent fat, and 15 to 20 percent protein. The guide is modeled after the USDA Food Guide Pyramid, with several noticeable differences.

1. *Dairy, eggs, other animal products, added fats, and sugar are in a category called "optional foods."* While animal products contain important nutrients, these nutrients can also be obtained from plant foods and fortified plant-based foods. Of course, plant foods offer tremendous advantages, as they are low in saturated fat, cholesterol-free, and brimming with the protective phytochemicals and fiber that are missing from animal foods. Fat and sugar are also optional, as they can be obtained from whole foods such as nuts, seeds, and fruits, which are infinitely more valuable to health.

2. *There are five food groups that are necessary components of a nutritious plant-based diet—vegetables, grains, legumes, fruits, and nuts and seeds.* While some would question the need for nuts and seeds, these are very important foods in plant-based diets. They are primary sources of essential fatty acids, vitamin E, and several trace minerals.

3. *Starchy vegetables are included in the grains group.* While there are important differences between starchy vegetables and whole grains, their carbohydrate content is very similar. Including them in the same group allows for greater consistency of carbohydrate intake.

The Plant-Based Food Guide for People with Diabetes—A Closer Look

The serving sizes for foods in each of the plant-based food groups are provided in table 5.1. The serving sizes for foods in the "optional foods" category are provided in table 5.2. In addition, servings for each of three levels of calories are indicated (1,500, 1,800, and 2,100 calories). While these three levels will not meet everyone's needs, they will promote a weight loss of 1 to 2 pounds a week (or allow for weight maintenance) in most people with type 2 diabetes. The following guidelines will help you to determine what level of calories is best for you.

- 1,500 calories—weight loss in most women and small or inactive men; weight maintenance in small, inactive, and/or senior women.
- 1,800 calories—weight loss in most men and active or larger women; weight maintenance for most women and small, inactive, and/or senior men.
- 2,100 calories—weight loss in active or large men; weight maintenance in most men and large or active women.

You may be thinking that this seems a little reminiscent of exchange systems, and indeed the food guide can be used in a similar way. It is very flexible in that it can simply provide direction in planning a nutritionally adequate diet, or it can be followed more rigidly as a plant-based version of the exchange system. Most people adopting a plant-based diet find that if they need the more rigid numbers and portion sizes, these are generally only required in the early stages of the transition. After this time, they can generally manage without any such aids. Details for use as an exchange system are provided at the end of the chapter and titled "Notes for Dietitians."

YOUR DAILY FOOD CHOICES

The Plant-Based Food Guide for People with Diabetes is a tool meant to assist you in designing a nutritious, balanced diet. Refer back to the information on various nutrients provided in chapters 3 and 4 to help with your menu selections. Now let's consider your choices within each food group.

Grains and Starchy Vegetables (6 to 11 servings)

Whole grains are key sources of B-vitamins, trace minerals, and vitamin E. Your best choices are intact grains such as kamut, spelt or wheat berries, oat groats, barley, brown rice, and quinoa. Your next best choices are those in which the grains have been processed in some way, but without removing the bran or germ. Examples would include oatmeal, shredded wheat, whole grain breads and cereals, whole grain pasta, and whole grain crackers. Less desirable choices include all refined products; limit these to not more than two servings per day. Starchy vegetables are good sources of vitamin C, vitamin A, and B vitamins. (Orange and yellow vegetables contain much higher levels of vitamin A in the form of beta-carotene.) All types of potatoes, corn, winter squash, and plantain are good choices. Keep the skin on the potatoes to increase both nutrients and fiber content.

Vegetables (4 or more servings)

Vegetables are the most nutrient-dense foods in the diet. That means they provide the highest levels of nutrients for the fewest number of calories. Vegetables are rich sources of vitamins A, C, and K, several B vitamins, and a range of minerals. They are also phytochemical powerhouses. While variety is the real key to maximizing the benefits from these foods, dark green leafy vegetables definitely stand out as being especially protective. Make vegetables the central part of your meals for at least one or two meals each day. Include both cooked and raw vegetables where possible. Keep washed, cut-up vegetables in the fridge as handy snacks.

Legumes (4 to 6 servings)

Legumes are important sources of protein, iron, and zinc. They also contain a wealth of B vitamins, trace minerals, and some calcium. For many people, increasing legume consumption is one of the toughest dietary adjustments they make. Most of us didn't grow up eating many legumes, so we just don't know what to do with them. In addition, people may initially find legumes hard to digest and complain of bloating and gas.

The best way to incorporate legumes into the diet is to start small. Add them to soups, stews, pasta sauces, salads, and stir-fries. This gradual increase in legume use will help your system adjust to the increased fiber intake, causing fewer digestive difficulties. Smaller legumes, such as French lentils and split peas, may be easiest to digest. While you are slowly increasing bean consumption, use some tofu and tempeh, foods which have been used in Asia for centuries, as well as some of the new veggie "meats." Once you get comfortable with legumes, try many of the wonderful ethnic recipes that contain larger amounts of beans. Experiment with bean patties and roasts, dips, and sauces.

Fruits (2 to 5 servings)

Fruits are good sources of vitamins A and C, folate, and several minerals. They are nature's treat and the very best way to satisfy your sweet tooth. Fresh fruits are a better option than fruit juices, as they provide greater satiety and more fiber and protective phytochemicals. They make great snacks and wonderful desserts. Use frozen fruits blended with a little soymilk or yogurt to make a delicious, low-fat, nutrition-packed "ice cream."

Nuts and Seeds (2 to 4 servings)

Nuts and seeds are rich sources of folate and vitamin E, a number of trace minerals (including selenium, copper, and magnesium), as well as essential

TABLE 5.1	Serving Sizes and Allowances for Plant-Based Food Groups

■ Food Group	Allowances	Servings per Calorie Level		
		1,500	**1,800**	**2,100**

Grains and Starchy Vegetables   6–11 servings   6   7   8
Select mainly whole, unprocessed grains and starchy vegetables prepared with little or no added fat.

serving size

Grains	
1 slice whole grain bread	1-1¼ cups (250-310 mL) puffed cereal
1½ cup (125 mL) cooked whole grain (rice, quinoa, kamut, barley, etc.)	½ cup (125 mL) cooked cereal
	⅓ cup (85 mL) muesli
½ whole grain bagel	½ cup (125 mL) pasta
½-¾ cup (125-185 mL) flaked cold cereal	3-4 whole grain crackers
	1 cup (250 mL) unbuttered popcorn

High-starch vegetables	¼ cup (60 mL) mashed sweet potato or yam
1 small potato	½ cup (125 mL) corn or 1 medium cob
½ small, baked sweet potato	1 cup (250 mL) winter squash
½ cup (125 mL) mashed potato	½ cup (125 mL) plantain

■ Food Group	Allowances	Servings per Calorie Level		
		1,500	**1,800**	**2,100**

Legumes   4–6 servings   4   5   6
Select at least 2 servings of beans, lentils, or split peas.

serving size

½ cup (125 mL) cooked beans, lentils, or split peas	1 cup (250 mL) soymilk
⅓ cup (85 mL) or 2½ oz (76 g) firm tofu or tempeh	1 cup (250 mL) cooked peas
	2 Tbsp. (30 mL) soy nuts
½ cup (125 mL) or 4⅓ oz (124 g) medium tofu	2 oz. (57 g) seitan
	2 oz. (57 g) veggie "meat"

■ Food Group	Allowances	Servings per Calorie Level		
		1,500	1,800	2,100

Vegetables
(Includes all vegetables except those in
the Grains and Starchy Vegetables Group)
Eat generous portions of a variety of vegetables.

4 or more servings   4 or more servings
for all calorie levels

serving size

1 cup (250 mL) raw vegetables   ½ cup (125 mL) vegetable juices
½ cup (125 mL) cooked vegetables

■ Food Group	Allowances	Servings per Calorie Level		
		1,500	1,800	2,100
Fruits	2–5 servings	3	4	5

Select mainly whole fresh fruits rather than fruit juices or canned or cooked fruits.

serving size

1 large kiwi, tangerine, or peach

1 medium orange, grapefruit, or nectarine

1 small apple or banana

½ large mango or pear

1 cup (250 mL) berries, papaya, or melon

10 large grapes (15-20 small)

4 small apricots

2 plums or fresh figs

½ cup (125 mL) applesauce or cooked
or canned fruit

¾ cup (185 mL) fresh pineapple or
grapefruit sections

3 Tbsp. (45 mL) dried fruit

½ cup (125 mL) fruit juice, most

⅓ cup (83 mL) prune juice

■ Food Group	Allowances	Servings per Calorie Level		
		1,500	1,800	2,100
Nuts and Seeds	2–5 servings	2½	3	3½

Select nuts and seeds without added fat or salt.

serving size

1 Tbsp. (15 mL) nut or seed butter

⅔ oz. (19 g) nuts or seeds (2 heaping Tbsp.)

⅓ whole avocado

fatty acids. They also contain high levels of the amino acid arginine, which is converted in the body to nitric oxide, a chemical that helps to dilate blood vessels, helping improve blood flow. Adding nuts and seeds to the diet is a snap. Throw them in a stir-fry, on a salad, or in your breakfast cereal. Remember that nuts and seeds are very-high-fat foods and should be used in moderate amounts.

You may be surprised to see that avocados are in the nut and seed group. Nutritionally speaking, avocados more closely resemble nuts and seeds than they do fruits. Avocados provide similar amounts of fat and carbohydrate, although slightly less protein, than nuts and seeds, however they are higher in protein than other fruits.

One serving of nuts and seeds provides, on average, 9 grams of fat and 4 grams each of protein and carbohydrates. One serving of avocado (one-third of the fruit) provides about 10 grams of fat, 5 grams carbohydrate, and almost 2 grams of protein. (The larger, smooth-skinned Florida avocados are lower in fat and higher in protein and carbohydrate than the smaller Haas or California avocados.)

While two to four servings may seem like a lot, this is your "fat allowance." Using nuts, seeds, and avocados is the very best way to consume fat, because it comes packaged with so many protective dietary components. If you want to use concentrated fats and oils, they will replace nut and seed servings. One nut and seed serving has about 9 grams of fat and 110 calories, while one fats and oils serving has only 5 grams of fat and 45 calories. Thus, two fats and oils will replace one nuts and seeds serving. You may replace some, but not all, of your nut and seed servings with concentrated fats and oils. At least one serving of nuts and seeds must remain!

Dairy Products (0 to 2 servings)

Dairy products provide protein, calcium, riboflavin, vitamins A and D, and several other minerals. While dairy products are not essential foods, they are a significant part of the diet for many people. The reason we limit total dairy intake is because we do not want dairy products to displace high-fiber, phytochemical-rich plant foods. If you do use dairy products, select those that are fat-free or at least low in fat (preferably one percent or less), as dairy fat is highly saturated. Your best choices are skim milk, skim milk yogurt, and low-fat cottage cheese. Dairy products will replace one to two legume servings (1 dairy serving = 1 legume serving). At least two legume servings must remain, including one serving of beans.

Eggs and Other Animal Products
(0 to 2 servings)

Eggs and other animal products are rich sources of protein, iron, and zinc. We include these in our plant-based food guide to allow choices for individuals in transition to a vegetarian diet or for those who use some animal products. If you do eat these foods, your best choices are omega-3-rich eggs and fish. If using any other animal products, choose only very lean items. Avoid processed meats of any kind. If using one to two servings of eggs and other animal products, they replace legumes (1 animal protein food = 1 legume). At least two legume servings must remain, with beans being the preferred option. Eggs and other animal products contain negligible amounts of carbohydrates, thus selecting beans, the highest carbohydrate foods in the legume group, helps to hold carbohydrate intake constant.

Fats and Oils (0 to 4 servings)

Concentrated fats and oils are not a necessary part of the diet. However, they can add value both in taste and nutrition, if well selected. For example, adding a little oil to a salad considerably enhances the nutrient and phytochemical absorption of the vegetables. If you do use some fats and oils, select unrefined, mechanically pressed, organic oils. In regular supermarkets, extra-virgin olive oil is generally the only unrefined oil available. The high monounsaturated fat content makes it an excellent choice. In natural food stores you will find other high-quality, fresh-pressed oils. (Those with high omega-3 content will be kept refrigerated.) Your best choices are flaxseed, canola, walnut, and hazelnut oil. Your primary cooking oil should be olive oil, high-oleic sunflower or safflower oil, or organic canola oil. If you use margarine, be sure it contains no hydrogenated fat (some palm oil is okay). Be very judicious in your use of added fats. Two fats and oils servings replace one nut and seed serving.

Sugars (0 to 3 servings)

For many years, sweets were considered an absolute no-no for people with diabetes. While there are still many good reasons not to overdo various sugars (first and foremost, their lack of nutritional value), occasional use of small amounts of sweeteners is completely reasonable. While there is some truth to the saying "sugar is sugar," some sweeteners are preferable in terms of nutrition and their effects on blood sugar. The only sweetener that offers any significant nutrition is blackstrap molasses, which is loaded with minerals,

TABLE 5.2 — Serving Sizes and Allowances for Optional Food Groups

■ Food Group	Allowances	Servings per Calorie Level		
		1,500	1,800	2,100
Dairy Products	0–2 servings	0–2	0–2	0–2

If used, select nonfat or low-fat dairy products. (If used, dairy, eggs, or other animal products may replace up to 3-4 servings of legumes, leaving <u>at least</u> 2 servings from the legume group. One serving of dairy or other animal products replaces 1 serving from the legumes group.

serving size

1 cup (250 mL) fat-free or low-fat milk   ¼ cup (60 mL) cottage cheese

½ cup (125 mL) fat-free evaporated milk   1 oz. (28 g) nonfat or low-fat cheese

¾ cup (185 mL) fat-free or low-fat yogurt

■ Food Group	Allowances	Servings per Calorie Level		
		1,500	1,800	2,100
Eggs and Other Animal Products	0–2 servings	0–1	0–2	0–2

If used, select mostly omega-3-rich eggs or fish.

serving size

1 large egg   1½ oz. (42 g) other flesh foods

3 oz. (83 g) fish

■ Food Group	Allowances	Servings per Calorie Level		
		1,500	1,800	2,100
Fats	0–4 servings	0–3	0–3	0–5

If used, select monounsaturated or omega-3-rich fats and oils. Avoid hydrogenated fats.
Fats will replace nut servings. Two fats replace 1 nut serving, leaving <u>at least</u> 1-2 servings of nuts and seeds each day.

serving size

1 tsp. (5 mL) oil   1 tsp. (5 mL) mayonnaise

1 tsp. (5 mL) nonhydrogenated margarine   1 Tbsp. (15 mL) reduced-fat mayonnaise

1 Tbsp. (15 mL) salad dressing

■ Food Group	Allowances	Servings per Calorie Level		
		1,500	1,800	2,100
Sugars	0–3 servings	0–1	0–2	0–3

If used, select mainly natural sweeteners such as blackstrap molasses, agave syrup, maple syrup, etc. Sugar may replace fruit servings, leaving <u>at least</u> 2 servings of fruit each day. One sugar equals 1 fruit serving.

serving size

1 Tbsp. (15 mL) sugar or liquid sugar— honey, corn syrup, agave syrup, brown rice syrup, molasses, sugar, brown sugar, etc.	1 Tbsp. (15 mL) jam or jelly ¾ oz. (21 g) candy ¾ cup (185 mL) sherbet

including hefty amounts of calcium and iron. Certain types of sugar also have less impact on blood sugar than others. Those that least affect blood sugar contain a higher proportion of fructose relative to glucose or sucrose. The newest "star" in the sugar world is agave nectar or syrup, which comes from a cactus-like plant. It has a very low glycemic index, as it is 90 percent fructose. (See chapter 6 for more information on sweets.) One sugar serving replaces one fruit. At least two fruit servings must remain.

Menu Planning—Make the Most of Your Meals

Now, let's move on to what really matters—the food you eat. In the next few pages you'll find meal and snack ideas for a full week. Use this as a guide to get started, then get creative! Preparing wonderful food can be as healing as it is nourishing. Always begin with high quality ingredients. Think whole, fresh, colorful foods. Make your food look appealing—a sprig of parsley, a carrot curl, or an edible flower can turn a plain dish into something special. Be adventurous; take a cooking class; try new foods and recipes!

Tables 5.3 through 5.6 provide menu suggestions for breakfast, lunch, dinner, and snacks. If you prefer to stick to three meals a day, your snack allowances can be incorporated into your meals. Each table outlines appropriate portions for each of three calorie levels: 1,500, 1,800, and 2,100. All the recipes for the suggested menus are provided on pages 201 to 251.

TABLE 5.3 — Breakfast Menu: 1,500, 1,800, and 2,100 Calorie Diets

Serving amounts are given for 1,500 calorie diets. Increased serving amounts for 1,800 and 2,100 calorie diets are listed below them. (Increased serving sizes for 1,800 calorie diets also apply to 2,100 calorie diets, unless otherwise specified.)
For total servings in each food group, see table 5.7.

■ Monday - 1,500 calorie diet	Food Groups
⅔ cup (165 mL) Whole Grain Breakfast Cereal, p. 203	2 grains*
2 Tbsp. (30 mL) walnuts	1 nut and seed
1 cup (250 mL) soymilk or skim milk	1 legume
1 cup (250 mL) blueberries	1 fruit
changes for 1,800/2,100 calorie diets (none)	

■ Tuesday - 1,500 calorie diet	Food Groups
½ cup (125 mL) Scrambled Tofu, p. 206	1½ legumes
2 slices veggie "back bacon"	½ legume
1 Irish-Style Scone, p. 212	1 grain, ½ nut and seed
1 grapefruit	1 fruit
changes for 1,800/2,100 calorie diets	
2 Irish-Style Scones, p. 212	2 grains, 1 nut and seed

■ Wednesday - 1,500 calorie diet	Food Groups
⅔ cup (165 mL) Morning Muesli, p. 205	2 grains, ½ nut and seed, ½ fruit
½ cup (125 mL) soymilk or skim milk	½ legume
½ cup (125 mL) strawberries	½ fruit
changes for 1,800/2,100 calorie diets	
1,800 calories	
1 cup (250 mL) Morning Muesli, p. 205	3 grains, ¾ nut and seed, ¾ fruit
1 cup (250 mL) soymilk or skim milk	1 legume
¾ cup (185 mL) strawberries	¾ fruit
2,100 calories	
1⅓ cup (333 mL) Morning Muesli, p. 205	4 grains, 1 nut and seed, 1 fruit
1½ cups (375 mL) soymilk or skim milk	1½ legumes
1 cup (250 mL) strawberries	1 fruit

■ Thursday - 1,500 calorie diet	Food Groups
1½ pieces French Toast, p. 204	1½ grains, ¾ nut and seed
2 slices veggie "ham"	5 legumes
½ cup (125 mL) Fresh Fruit Sauce, p. 207	½ fruit

changes for 1,800/2,100 calorie diets

1,800 calories

2 pieces French Toast, p. 204	2 grains, 1 nut and seed

2,100 calories

2 pieces French Toast, p. 204	2 grains, 1 nut and seed
1 cup (250 mL) Fresh Fruit Sauce, p. 207	1 fruit

■ Friday - 1,500 calorie diet — Food Groups

1½ slices Pumpernickel toast, p. 208	2 grains
1 Tbsp. (15 mL) almond butter	½ nut and seed
1 small banana	1 fruit
1 cup (250 mL) nondairy or skim milk	1 legume

changes for 1,800/2,100 calorie diets

2 slices Pumpernickel toast, p. 208	2 grains
2 Tbsp. (30 mL) almond butter	1 nut and seed

■ Saturday - 1,500 calorie diet — Food Groups

1 Applesauce-Raisin Muffin, p. 211	1 grain, ½ nut and seed, ½ fruit
1 cup (250 mL) soy or dairy yogurt	1 legume
½ cup (125 mL) fresh fruit salad	1 fruit

changes for 1,800/2,100 calorie diets

2,100 calories

1½ Applesauce-Raisin Muffins, p. 211	1½ grains, 1 nut and seed, 1 fruit
1½ cups (375 mL) soy or dairy yogurt	1½ legumes

■ Sunday - 1,500 calorie diet — Food Groups

1 Whole Grain Waffle, p. 202	2 grains, 1 nut and seed
¼ cup (60 mL) Fruit Syrup, p. 246	½ fruit
1 Tempeh Sausage, p. 231	1 legume

changes for 1,800/2,100 calorie diets

1,800 calories

2 Tempeh Sausages, p. 231	2 legumes

2,100 calories

1½ Whole Grain Waffles, p. 202	3 grains, 1½ nuts and seeds
½ cup (125 mL) Fruit Syrup, p. 246	1 fruit
2 Tempeh Sausages, p. 231	2 legumes

*"grains" will be used to indicate servings from the grains and starchy vegetables group.

TABLE 5.4 Lunch Menu - 1,500, 1,800, and 2,100 Calorie Diets

Serving amounts are given for 1,500 calorie diets. Increased serving amounts for 1,800 and 2,100 calorie diets are listed below them. (Increased serving sizes for 1,800 calorie diets also apply to 2,100 calorie diets, unless otherwise specified.)
For total servings in each food group, see table 5.7.

■ Monday - 1,500 calorie diet	Food Groups
½ cup (250 mL) Tofu Salad Delight, p. 229	1 legume, ½ nut and seed
3 Sesame Rye Thins, p. 209	1 grain*
1⅓ cups (333 mL) Marinated Vegetables, p. 237	1 vegetable
1 plum	½ fruit

changes for 1,800/2,100 calorie diets	
1,800 calories	
¾ cup (185 mL) Tofu Dip, p. 251	1½ legume, ¾ nut and seed
6 Sesame Rye Thins, p. 209	2 grains
2 plums	1 fruit
2,100 calories	
4 plums	2 fruit

■ Tuesday - 1,500 calorie diet	Food Groups
1¼ cups (310 mL) Black-Eyed Peas & Greens Soup, p. 220	1 legume, 1 vegetable
1 Herbed Muffin, p. 210	½ grain
1 cup (250 mL) Pickled Cucumbers, p. 215	1 vegetable, ⅔ nut and seed
½ cup (125 mL) cubed melon	½ fruit

changes for 1,800/2,100 calorie diets	
1,800 calories	
1 cup (250 mL) cubed melon	1 fruit
2,100 calories	
2½ cups (625 mL) Black-Eyed Peas & Greens Soup, p. 220	2 legumes, 2 vegetables

■ Wednesday - 1,500 calorie diet	Food Groups
1¼ cups (310 mL) Quinoa Salad, p. 227	1 grain, 1 vegetable, 1 legume, ½ nut and seed
1¼ cups (310 mL) Navy Bean Mushroom Soup, p. 218	1 legume, 1 vegetable
1 tangerine	1 fruit

changes for 1,800/2,100 calorie diets (none)	

*"grains" will be used to indicate servings from the grains and starchy vegetables group.

■ Thursday - 1,500 calorie diet	Food Groups
¼ cup (60 mL) Roasted Garlic Hummus, p. 249	½ legume, ½ nut and seed
one 6" whole-wheat pita bread	2 grains
1 cup or more (250 mL) raw vegetables	1 vegetable
¼ cup (60 mL) Cucumber-Mint Dip, p. 248	¼ nut and seed
changes for 1,800/2,100 calorie diets	
½ cup (125 mL) Roasted Garlic Hummus, p. 249	1 legume, 1 nut and seed

■ Friday - 1,500 calorie diet	Food Groups
¾ cup (185 mL) Sweet Potato Salad, p. 217	1½ grains, ½ nut and seed
1¼ cups (310 mL) Triple Bean Soup, p. 219	1½ legumes, ½ nut and seed, ½ vegetable
1¼ oz. (35 g) flavored firm tofu	½ legume
½ large mango	1 fruit
changes for 1,800/2,100 calorie diets	
1,800 calories	
2½ oz. (70 g) flavored firm tofu	1 legume
1 large mango	2 fruit
2,100 calories	
3¾ oz. (105 g) flavored firm tofu	1½ legumes

■ Saturday - 1,500 calorie diet	Food Groups
1 Barley Burger (with bun and condiments), p. 232	3 grains, ¾ nut and seed
½ Tbsp. (7 mL) low-fat mayonnaise	¼ nut and seed
2 slices veggie "back bacon" (for burger)	½ legume
2 cups (500 mL) Marinated Vegetables, p. 237	2 vegetables
changes for 1,800/2,100 calorie diets	
1 Tbsp. (15 mL) low-fat mayonnaise	½ nut and seed

■ Sunday - 1,500 calorie diet	Food Groups
1 cup (250 mL) Arugula & Garbanzo Bean Salad, p. 224	1 grain, 1 vegetable, ¾ legume, ½ nut and seed
½ slice Pumpernickel Bread, p. 208	½ grain
1 tsp. (5 mL) almond butter	⅓ nut and seed
1 medium kiwi	1 fruit
changes for 1,800/2,100 calorie diets	
1 slice Pumpernickel Bread, p. 208	1 grain
2 tsp. (10 mL) almond butter	⅔ nut and seed

| TABLE 5.5 | Dinner Menu - 1,500, 1,800, and 2,100 calorie diets |

Serving amounts are given for 1,500 calorie diets. Increased serving amounts for 1,800 and 2,100 calorie diets are listed below them. (Increased serving sizes for 1,800 calorie diets also apply to 2,100 calorie diets, unless otherwise specified.)
For total servings in each food group, see table 5.7.

■ Monday - 1,500 calorie diet	Food Groups
1½ cups (375 mL) Barley and Lentil Stew, p. 225	2 grains*, 1 vegetable, 1 legume
1 cup (250 mL) Fresh Spinach Salad, p. 216	1 vegetable, ½ nut and seed
⅓ cup (85 mL) Apple Crisp, p. 239	½ grain, ½ fruit, ⅓ nut and seed

changes for 1,800/2,100 calorie diets	
1,800 calories	
1½ cups (375 mL) Fresh Spinach Salad, p. 216	1½ vegetables, 1 nut and seed
⅔ cup (165 mL) Apple Crisp, p. 239	1 grain, 1 fruit, ¾ nut and seed
2,100 calories	
2¼ cups (560 mL) Barley and Lentil Stew, p. 225	3 grains, 1½ vegetables, 1½ legumes

■ Tuesday - 1,500 calorie diet	Food Groups
1½ cups (375 mL) Oven Baked Veggies, p. 222-23	1¼ legumes, 1 grain, 2 vegetables
⅔ cup (165 mL) Millet Pudding, p. 245	1 grain, ½ nut and seed
1 cup sliced strawberries	1 fruit

changes for 1,800/2,100 calorie diets	
1,800 calories	
2¼ cups (560 mL) Oven Baked Veggies, p. 222-23	2 legumes, 1½ grains, 3 vegetables
2,100 calories	
3 cups (750 mL) Oven Baked Veggies, p. 222-23	2½ legumes, 2 grains, 4 vegetables

■ Wednesday - 1,500 calorie diet	Food Groups
1¼ cups (310 mL) Gingered Garbanzo Beans, p. 235	1 legume, 2 vegetables
1 cup (250 mL) brown and wild rice	2 grains
2½ cups (625 mL) green salad with flax dressing	2 vegetables, 1 nut and seed
½ cup (125 mL) fresh fruit salad	1 fruit

changes for 1,800/2,100 calorie diets	
1,800 calories	
¾ cup (185 mL) fresh fruit salad	1½ fruits
2,100 calories	
2 cups (500 mL) Gingered Garbanzo Beans, p. 235	1½ legumes, 3 vegetables
1 cup (250 mL) fresh fruit salad	2 fruits

*"grains" will be used to indicate servings from the grains and starchy vegetables group.

■ Thursday - 1,500 calorie diet	**Food Groups**
1¼ cups (310 mL) Stuffed Zucchini, p. 221	1½ grains, 1 legume, 1 vegetable, 1 nut and seed
¾ cup (185 mL) Green Beans w/ Lemon, p. 234	1 vegetable, ½ nut and seed
1 Brenda's Date Cookie, p. 242	½ grain, ½ fruit, ¼ nut and seed

changes for 1,800/2,100 calorie diets

1,800 calories

1½ cups (375 mL) Green Beans w/ Lemon, p. 234	2 vegetables, 1 nut and seed
2 Brenda's Date Cookies, p. 242	1 grain, 1 fruit, ½ nut and seed

2,100 calories

2 cups (500 mL) Stuffed Zucchini, p. 221	2¼ grains, 1½ legumes, 1½ vegetables, 1½ nuts and seeds

■ Friday - 1,500 calorie diet	**Food Groups**
1½ cups (375 mL) Lentil Pie, p. 226	1 legume, 1 grain, 1 vegetable, ¼ nut/seed
½ cup (125 mL) Spicy Cabbage, p. 236	1 vegetable, ½ nut and seed
1 Treatie Ball, p. 244	½ grain, ½ nut and seed

changes for 1,800/2,100 calorie diets

1,800 calories

¾ cup (185 mL) Spicy Cabbage, p. 236	1½ vegetables, ¾ nut and seed

2,100 calories

2¼ cups (560 mL) Lentil Pie, p. 226	1½ legumes, 1½ grains, 1½ vegetables, ⅓ nut and seed
2 Treatie Balls, p. 244	1 grain, 1 nut and seed

■ Saturday - 1,500 calorie diet	**Food Groups**
1⅔ cups (415 mL) Polenta-Tempeh Bake, p. 228-29	1 legume, 1 grain, 1 vegetable
1⅓ cups (333 mL) Red Cabbage Slaw, p. 213	2 vegetables, 1 nut and seed
1 cup (250 mL) Iced Fruit Cream, p. 243	2 fruits, 1 legume

changes for 1,800/2,100 calorie diets

1,800 calories

2½ cups (625 mL) Polenta Tempeh Bake, p. 228-29	1½ legumes, 1½ grains, 1½ vegetables

2,100 calories

2 cups (500 mL) Red Cabbage Slaw, p. 213	2 vegetables, 1 nut and seed
1½ cups (375 mL) Iced Fruit Cream, p. 243	3 fruits, 1½ legumes

■ Sunday - 1,500 calorie diet	**Food Groups**
1 Vegetable Skewer, p. 230	1⅓ legumes, ½ nut/seed, 2 vegetables
¼ cup (60 mL) brown rice	½ grain
¾ cup (185 mL) Baked Squash Casserole, p. 233	1 grain, 1 fruit
1/10 fruit pie	1 grain, 1 fruit, ¼ nut and seed

changes for 1,800/2,100 calorie diets (none)

TABLE 5.6	Snack Menu - 1,500, 1,800, and 2,100 calorie diets

Serving amounts are given for 1,500 calorie diets. Increased serving amounts for 1,800 and 2,100 calorie diets are listed below them. (Increased serving sizes for 1,800 calorie diets also apply to 2,100 calorie diets, unless otherwise specified.)
For total servings in each food group, see table 5.7.

■ Monday - 1,500 calorie diet	Food Groups
1 fresh orange	1 fruit
2 Tbsp. (30 mL) soy nuts	1 legume
1 cup (250 mL) or more raw vegetables	1 vegetable
changes for 1,800/2,100 calorie diets (none)	

■ Tuesday - 1,500 calorie diet	Food Groups
2 wheatless cookies	1½ grains*
2 Tbsp. (30 mL) Tamari Roasted Almonds, p. 247	1 nut and seed
1 small fresh peach	½ fruit
changes for 1,800/2,100 calorie diets	
1,800 calories	
3 Tbsp. (45 mL) Tamari Roasted Almonds, p. 247	1½ nuts and seeds
1 large fresh peach	1 fruit
2,100 calories	
¼ cup. (60 mL) Tamari Roasted Almonds, p. 247	2 nuts and seeds
2 large fresh peaches	2 fruits

■ Wednesday - 1,500 calorie diet	Food Groups
2 rice cakes	1 grain
2 slices veggie "salami"	½ legume
½ cup (125 mL) Pickled Cucumbers, p. 215	1 vegetable
1 Tbsp. (15 mL) pumpkin seeds	½ nut and seed
changes for 1,800/2,100 calorie diets	
1,800 calories	
4 slices veggie "salami"	1 legume
1½ Tbsp. (22 mL) pumpkin seeds	¾ nut and seed
2,100 calories	
2 Tbsp. (30 mL) pumpkin seeds	1 nut and seed

*"grains" will be used to indicate servings from the grains and starchy vegetables group.

■ Thursday - 1,500 calorie diet	Food Groups
1 cup (250 mL) Iced Fruit Cream, p. 243	2 fruits, 1 legume
1 cup (250 mL) or more raw vegetables	1 vegetable
changes for 1,800/2,100 calorie diets	
1,800 calories	
1½ cups (375 mL) Iced Fruit Cream, p. 243	3 fruits, 1½ legumes

■ Friday - 1,500 calorie diet	Food Groups
2 cups (500 mL) Popcorn, p. 250	1 grain
14 fresh cherries	1 fruit
1 piece Celery Snacks, p. 247	¼ nut and seed
changes for 1,800/2,100 calorie diets	
1,800 calories	
2 pieces Celery Snacks, p. 247	½ nut and seed

■ Saturday - 1,500 calorie diet	Food Groups
3 Sesame Rye Thins, p. 209	1 grain
1 Tbsp. (15 mL) soynut butter	½ legume
changes for 1,800/2,100 calorie diets	
6 Sesame Rye Thins, p. 209	2 grains
1 plum	½ fruit

■ Sunday - 1,500 calorie diet	Food Groups
1 cup (250 mL) fruit smoothie with soymilk (1 cup frozen fruit for each cup soymilk)	1 legume, 1 fruit
8 Tamari Roasted Almonds, p. 247	½ nut and seed
1 cup (250 mL) or more raw vegetables	1 vegetable
changes for 1,800/2,100 calorie diets	
1,800 calories	
16 Tamari Roasted Almonds, p. 247	1 nut and seed
2,100 calories	
2 cups (500 mL) fruit smoothie with soymilk (1 cup frozen fruit for each cup soymilk)	2 legumes, 1 fruit

TABLE 5.7	Daily Intakes for Each Food Group					
CALORIE LEVEL	GRAINS & STARCHY VEGETABLES	LEGUMES	VEGETABLES	FRUITS	NUTS & SEEDS	ACTUAL CALORIES
Monday						
1,500	5½	4	4	3	2⅓	1,564
1,800	7	5	4½	4	3½	1,817
2,100	8	6	5	5	3¾	2,113
Tuesday						
1,500	6	4¼	5	3	2⅔	1,501
1,800	7½	5	6	4	3⅔	1,760
2,100	8	6	7	5	4⅙	2,113
Wednesday						
1,500	6	4	7	3	2½	1,537
1,800	7	5	7	4	3	1,737
2,100	8	6	8	5	3½	2,045
Thursday						
1,500	5½	3	4	3	3¼	1,509
1,800	6½	4	5	4½	4¾	1,858
2,100	7¼	4½	5½	5	5¼	2,121
Friday						
1,500	6	4	3	3	3	1,533
1,800	7	4½	4	4	4	1,833
2,100	8	5½	4	4	4½	2,116
Saturday						
1,500	6	4	5	3½	2½	1,492
1,800	7½	5	5½	4¼	3	1,844
2,100	8	6	5½	5½	3¼	2,096
Sunday						
1,500	6	4	4	3½	3	1,551
1,800	7	5	4	3½	4	1,839
2,100	8	5	4	4	4½	2,111
Suggested Intakes for Each Calorie Level						
1,500	6	4	4 or more	3	2½	
1,800	7	5	4 or more	4	3	
2,100	8	6	4 or more	5	3½	

TABLE 5.8   Nutrients of Concern

Calcium	19-50 yrs: 1,000 mg/day	50+ years: 1,200 mg/day

One serving = 120-150 mg of calcium:

½ cup (125 mL) calcium fortified nondairy milk

½ cup (125 mL) cow's milk

⅓ cup (85 mL) yogurt

¼ cup (60 mL) calcium-set tofu

½ cup (125 mL) calcium-fortified orange juice

1 cup (250 mL) cooked or 2 cups raw calcium-rich greens (kale, collards, broccoli, Chinese greens)

1 cup (250 mL) cottage cheese

1 oz. (28 g) low-fat cheese

⅓ cup (85 mL) or 1.7 oz (48 g) almonds

3 Tbsp. (45 mL) almond butter

1 cup (250 mL) calcium-rich beans (soy, white, navy, black turtle, Great Northern)

1 Tbsp. (15 mL) blackstrap molasses

5 figs

¼ cup hijiki seaweed

Special considerations

Getting enough calcium can be a challenge. In our culture, dairy products are the most well-recognized sources. However, there are also many plant sources, as well as a number of calcium-fortified foods. It is important to ensure your daily diet provides sufficient calcium. Choose at least six servings of calcium-rich foods if you are 19 to 50 years of age and eight servings if you are over 50 years of age. If eating fewer servings, take a calcium supplement.

Vitamin D	19-50 yrs : 5 mcg	51-70 yrs: 10 mcg	70+ yrs: 15 mcg

Sunshine: 10-15 minutes of warm sunlight on face and forearms for light- skinned people (3-6 times more for people with darker skin)

Foods: fortified products including cow's milk, nondairy beverages, margarines and cereals are our primary vitamin D sources. Check labels for amounts.

Special considerations

People at risk for vitamin D deficiency are those who have limited access to warm sunshine and/or those who do not use fortified with vitamin D. In these cases, a supplement should be taken.

Vitamin B$_{12}$	Adults: 2.4 mcg

Fortified foods:	Some breakfast cereals
Fortified nondairy beverages	Some veggie "meats"
Red Star Vegetarian Support Formula	**Animal foods:**
Nutritional Yeast (not all Red Star yeast is fortified)	Dairy, eggs, and meat

Special considerations

Vitamin B$_{12}$ in fortified foods or supplements is essential for vegans. As we get older, our ability to utilize the B$_{12}$ in animal products is reduced. Thus, vegans, along with anyone over 50 years of age, should include B$_{12}$ in the form of fortified foods or a supplement.

Omega-3 Fatty Acids	3-5 grams per day

Plant sources
Flaxseed, hempseed, canola oil, soy foods, walnuts, dark greens, sea vegetables.

Animal sources
Fish, eggs (especially omega-3-rich varieties)

Special considerations

Omega-3 fatty acids are unstable, so foods rich in these fats should be refrigerated or frozen. Supplementary DHA (microalgae) can be obtained from supplements (see page 74).

TABLE 5.9 Energy and Energy-Giving Nutrients of Plant-Based Foods

FOOD LIST	ENERGY (kcal)	CHO (g)	PROTEIN (g)	FAT (g)
Grains and Starchy Vegetables	80	15	3	1
Vegetables	25	5	2	0
Legumes	110	12	9	3
Fruits	65	15	1	0
Nuts and Seeds	110	4	4	9

Notes: These figures are based on one serving of food from each food group. Serving sizes are shown in table 5.1. There is some variation in the total energy and energy-giving nutrient content of the foods in each of these groups. The group with the greatest variation is the legume group. Thus, the values for the legume group are based on an average of a mix of foods from this group. Table 5.10 on page 122 provides a list of selected items in the legume group, and the approximate energy, carbohydrate, protein, and fat content of these foods, per serving.

NOTES FOR DIETITIANS

s a dietitian, you will need a little more information about the Plant-Based Food Guide for People with Diabetes, particularly if you wish to use this guide as a modified exchange program.

Like the conventional exchange system, the plant-based system has some limitations; however, it offers numerous advantages. This system provides patients with an excellent balance of energy-giving nutrients and optimal intakes of nutrients, fiber, and other protective dietary components. It also minimizes saturated fat, trans fatty acids, cholesterol, refined carbohydrates, and other potentially damaging dietary components.

Table 5.9 provides the relative amounts of energy, carbohydrates, protein, and fat for foods in each food group below the "optional" line. Optional foods are discussed on the following pages.

Optional Foods

In this guide we allow for the use of dairy products, animal protein foods, and concentrated fats and sugars, but these foods are considered optional. Thus, we do not include them in the "allowances" (see tables 5.1 and 5.2) set up for various calorie levels. However, these foods may replace foods from the plant food groups (up to a specified limit, ensuring the minimum number of servings of plant foods necessary to produce the desirable therapeutic benefits). While these substitutions will cause some changes in intakes of energy-giving nutrients, the overall effects on carbohydrate load are not significant. Let's consider each of the optional groups.

Dairy Products

If dairy products are used, they replace up to two servings from the legumes group, leaving at least two servings of legumes. (For example, if a person is allotted four servings of legumes, two servings of legumes can be replaced by dairy products.) We advocate the use of low-fat or nonfat dairy products only. Thus, the total energy content of one serving would be in the 90 to 110 calorie range. In one serving of milk (1 cup/250 mL) there are 12 grams carbohydrate, 8 grams protein, and 0 to 3 grams of fat. Thus, dairy products replace foods in the legume group very well, in terms of both calories and energy-giving nutrients.

Eggs and Other Animal Products

This group includes eggs, fish, and other lean flesh foods. If used, these foods may replace up to two servings of legumes, as long as two legumes remain.

TABLE 5.10 Energy and Energy-Giving Nutrients of Selected Legumes				
	CALORIES	CHO	PROTEIN	FAT
Beans, most, ½ cup (125 mL)	115	20	7	1
Beans, soy, ½ cup (125 mL)	146	9	14	7
Tofu, firm or tempeh ⅓ cup/2.5 oz (85 mL/76 g)	110	3	12	7
Tofu, medium, ½ cup/4.4 oz (125 mL/124 g)	94	2	10	6
Peas, 1 cup (250 mL)	126	22	8	0
Soymilk, 1 cup (250 mL)	80	6	6	3
Soynuts, 2 tbsp (30 mL)	96	8	7	5
Veggie "meats," 2 oz (57 g)* (e.g. Yves deli slices)	80	6	14	0

*Note: Some veggie "meats" are higher in fat. Check labels.

(For example, if a person is allotted four servings of legumes, two of the legume servings can be replaced by two servings of eggs and other animal products.) When only two servings of legumes remain, beans are the preferred option. This will keep total carbohydrate intake in check, as well as ensuring adequate dietary fiber intake. (Eggs and other animal products contain virtually no carbohydrate, while beans have the most carbohydrate in the legume group.) The allowances in this group are 1 large egg, 3 ounces (85 g) of fish, and 1½ ounces (43 g) of lean meat.

Fats and Oils
If concentrated fats and oils are used, two servings will replace one nut and seed serving. At least one serving of nuts and seeds should remain. (For example, if a person is allotted three servings of nuts and seeds, they can replace two of the nuts and seeds with four servings of fats and oils.) One fats and oils choice provides about five grams of fat and no protein or carbohydrate. Two servings of fats and oils provide about 90 calories and 10 grams of fat, while one serving of nuts and seeds provide about 110 calories and 9 grams of fat.

Sugars
If sugars are used, they replace fruit servings. One serving of sugar replaces one serving of fruit, but at least two servings of fruit must remain. (For example, if a person is allotted four servings of fruit, they may replace two of those servings with jam, maple syrup, or other sugars.) Sugars provide about 12 to 15 grams of carbohydrates per serving.

CHAPTER 6

Making Sense of Sweets

The attraction to sweet foods is a well-recognized part of our survival apparatus. Historically, foods with a sweet taste were those that were generally safe to eat. Our primate cousins, having lost the ability to manufacture vitamin C, sought out sweet fruits as a source of ascorbic acid, or vitamin C. For example, researchers in the field have documented the importance to chimpanzees of communicating to each other where the available sweet fruit is located. However, this natural affinity for sweet flavors is more of an obstacle to continued good health in the face of today's unlimited quantities of concentrated sugars in packaged and processed foods, and widespread overconsumption of sweet beverages, such as sodas and fruit juices. It is estimated that the average North American family of four consumes two to five pounds of sugar weekly. Concern about the dangers of excess refined sugars in the diet has paved the way for a lucrative market for alternative sweeteners. Imagine getting the highly desirable sweet taste without calories or enjoying the sweet taste without any adverse health consequences. Marketing wizards are having a field day.

Endless Options

Sweeteners can be divided into two categories—nutritive and nonnutritive. Nutritive sweeteners provide energy or calories (about 4 calories per gram, like other carbohydrates or protein). These include sugar, brown sugar, honey, corn syrup, and other common sugars. Alternative nutritive sweeteners include turbinado sugar, raw sugar, barley malt, brown rice syrup, Sucanat, agave syrup, and others. All of these solid and liquid sugars taste sweet because of the presence of glucose, fructose, and/or sucrose. Another group of nutritive sweeteners are the sugar alcohols or polyols, including mannitol, sorbitol, xylitol, erythritol, isomalt, lactitol, maltitol, and hydrogenated starch hydrolysates. Sugar alcohols are found naturally in berries, apples, plums, and other foods, but are also produced commercially from carbohydrates for use in sugar-free candies, cookies, and chewing gum.

Nonnutritive sweeteners, also called sugar substitutes or artificial sweeteners, provide a sweet taste but are not a significant source of calories. In addition, these sweeteners do not affect blood sugar levels. There are currently four sugar substitutes approved for use in the United States: saccharin, aspartame, acesulfame potassium (acesulfame K or ace K), and sucralose. In Canada, all of those permitted in the U.S. are approved, plus cyclamates. There is one other sweetener that is technically nonnutritive, but is not an "artificial" sweetener. This is the herb stevia. At the present time, stevia is permitted for use only as a dietary supplement in both the U.S. and Canada.

NONNUTRITIVE SWEETENERS
TOO GOOD TO BE TRUE?

The safety of nonnutritive sweeteners is a topic of tremendous ongoing controversy. The national diabetes and dietetic associations, as well as U.S. and Canadian government agencies, all agree that several nonnutritive sweeteners are safe when used in moderate amounts. However, not all experts echo that sentiment, some claiming that these products are downright dangerous.

Saccharin   Saccharin has been around for well over one hundred years and is approved for use in over one hundred countries. While originally included on the "generally recognized as safe" (GRAS) list, it was removed in 1977 due to concerns about a link to cancer in lab rats. All products containing saccharin were required to carry the following warning: "Use of this product may be hazardous to your health. This product contains saccharin which has been determined to cause cancer in laboratory animals." Since 1981, saccharin has been listed as an "anticipated" human carcinogen in the U.S. However, several studies of high users (e.g., persons with diabetes) failed to support an association between saccharin and cancer, so in 2001 the decision against saccharin was reversed and warnings on labels were no longer required.

Prominent health organizations, including the American Cancer Society, the American Medical Association, and the American Dietetics Association also support saccharin's safety. Among the voices against lifting the saccharin warning on labels has been the nonprofit food watchdog agency Center for Science in the Public Interest (CSPI) and the National Institutes of Health (NIH). CSPI charged that the favorable evaluation of saccharin was "unscientific" because about half of the twenty-six-member review committee was tied to industry. They added that the committee inappropriately ignored or dismissed all the evidence that saccharin caused cancer in humans or animals, except for the well-accepted link to bladder cancer in male rats. CSPI's position is that the evidence on saccharin is mixed, and it should continue to be considered a potential carcinogen until further evidence suggests otherwise. Likewise, a panel representing the NIH recommended against removing saccharin from the list of chemicals that may possibly cause cancer in humans. The rationale was based on evidence of increased cancer risk among male rats fed saccharin. In addition, panel members felt that they could not ignore studies suggesting an increased risk among some categories of people, such as men who are heavy smokers.

> Verdict: While small amounts of saccharin are not likely to be a problem, regular use is questionable, and there are certainly better options.

Aspartame   Aspartame has been approved for use in over one hundred countries. It is arguably the most popular nonnutritive sweetener and also the most controversial. In 1981, the U.S. Food and Drug Administration (FDA) approved aspartame for use as a tabletop sweetener, and for use in cold breakfast cereal, gelatins, pudding, chewing gum, and carbonated beverages. In 1996, following numerous scientific evaluations, the FDA gave its stamp of approval for aspartame to be used as a general-purpose sweetener for all foods and beverages. Aspartame is considered one of the most highly tested food ingredients on the market. It is reported that prior to its approval, over one hundred scientific studies affirmed its safety. These studies were conducted in both animals and humans, including healthy adults and children, people with diabetes, and lactating women. The safety of aspartame has been affirmed not only by the FDA, but also by numerous health organizations such as the Joint Expert Committee on Food Additives (JECFA—the scientific advisory body to the World Health Organization and the Food and Agriculture Organization), the Scientific Committee for Food of the European Union, the Centers for Disease Control (CDC), the American Medical Association, the American Academy of Pediatrics, the American Dietetic Association, the American Diabetes Association, and the American Academy of Family Physicians. While aspartame gets the overwhelming stamp of approval from government agencies and health organizations around the world, the safety of aspartame has been strongly challenged. Doing a simple Internet search for "dangers of aspartame," will give you some idea of the extent of the controversy.

Anti-aspartame activists claim that "aspartame kills," and that complaints against aspartame constitute 75 percent of all additive-related complaints to the FDA department of consumer complaints. They warn consumers that methanol (wood alcohol) makes up 10 percent of aspartame and is highly toxic. While they admit that methanol is also found in some fruits and vegetables, they add that it is never found in natural foods without ethanol and pectin. Ethanol and pectin are said to act as antidotes to methanol, preventing it from being metabolized into formaldehyde and formic acid, both deadly toxins. They remind consumers that aspartame contains no ethanol or pectin; therefore, the methanol is converted to these deadly toxins. The anti-aspartame contingent also points out that while phenylalanine and aspartic acid (the amino acids in aspartame) are also found in natural foods, they are always a part of long chains of amino acids that are bound together to make protein molecules. They add that when consumed separately from other amino acids, the two amino acids in aspartame quickly enter the brain and central nervous system and act as a potent neurotoxin. Diseases and disorders said to be caused by aspartame include arthritis, ALS (Lou Gehrig's disease), Alzheimer's disease, cancer (especially brain cancer), confusion, diabetes, depression, dizziness, epilepsy, heart disease, birth defects, blurred vision, blindness, cataracts, fibromyalgia, headaches, lupus, multiple sclerosis, Parkinson's disease, and many, many others.

This is all terribly confusing for the average consumer. Who is telling the truth, the FDA and national governments who we pay to protect us or the seemingly fanatic anti-aspartame activists? It would seem like such a straightforward choice. Yet, even if there is a grain of truth to what the "extremists" are saying, it does present some cause for concern. In our experience, aspartame is not likely a deadly poison, but it does appear to cause adverse reactions in many people. For this reason, we would suggest limiting its use or eliminating it altogether.

Verdict: If you must use artificial sweeteners, this is not your best option. Remember, it is everywhere—more than six thousand products contain this sweetener!

Sucralose   The FDA, the Joint Food and Agricultural Organization of the World Health Organization, the American Council on Science and Health, and the Health Protection Branch of Health Canada all vouch for the safety of sucralose. Prior to giving its approval, the FDA examined over one hundred safety studies and forty environmental studies conducted over a twenty-year period. Overall, sucralose has generated relatively little negative press. However, as with most products, we managed to find a few outspoken critics. They claim that sucralose causes "shrunken thymus glands" and enlarged kidneys and liver. They also express concern about the presence of chlorine in the sweetener, stating that consuming sucralose may be like ingesting tiny amounts of chlorinated pesticides.

Verdict: Based on research to date, sucralose appears to be the safest of the "artificial" nonnutritive sweeteners. However, sucralose is a highly processed sweetener, so if you are aiming for a minimally processed diet, you'll want to limit your intake.

Acesulfame K   Though lesser known, acesulfame K (K stands for potassium) was approved in the U.S. for addition to foods in 1988, alcoholic beverages in 1995, and soft drinks in 1998. The Joint Expert Committee on Food Additives also reviewed relevant literature and concluded that it is safe. While numerous governments and regulatory agencies agree acesulfame K poses little risk, many other experts argue that its safety is questionable at best.

Some of the most vocal opposition has come from CSPI. It expressed serious concern that acesulfame K may be a potential carcinogen. In June 1995, CSPI filed a protest with the FDA, saying that the sweetener's safety had not been appropriately confirmed in long-term studies. According to CSPI, tests done on acesulfame K "followed inadequate protocols, which are greatly at variance with current standards for test design, execution and reporting required for the National Toxicology Program's bioassays." Numerous leading cancer experts provided CSPI with statements of support to assist in their efforts to get this sweetener reassessed.

> Verdict: While insignificant exposure to acesulfame K is unlikely a danger, higher intakes (for example, frequently drinking soda that is sweetened with acesulfame K) may be problematic. There are better options!

Cyclamate Cyclamate is the one nonnutritive sweetener that is permitted for use in Canada, but not in the U.S. In Canada, cyclamate can be sold only as a table sweetener, but in several European countries, cyclamate is widely used in beverages and food products. In 1969, the U.S. banned cyclamate on the basis of animal studies that linked cyclamate use to bladder cancer in rats and deformities in chick embryos (similar to those observed in babies of women who had used thalidomide to reduce severe morning sickness in the late 1950s). Some evidence also suggested that cyclamate might damage chromosomes in the cells of both animals and human beings, resulting in long-term adverse health consequences. Since then, however, two dozen long-term cancer studies, more than seventy experiments looking for genetic damage, and exhaustive reviews of the National Cancer Institute, the National Academy of Sciences, and the Joint Expert Committee on Food Additives have failed to confirm any significant adverse affects. In the U.S., a petition for cyclamate reapproval is currently under review by the FDA, and it is expected that it will soon be back in the food supply.

> Verdict: It appears that cyclamate may not be as damaging as was once thought, and the likelihood that it will be permitted for use in the U.S. once again is strong. However, like other artificial sweeteners, it may not be innocuous. So, while you needn't fret about trace amounts in foods, we wouldn't suggest regular, heavy use.

THE BOTTOM LINE

Artificial sweeteners are not "health foods." There is no evidence at all that they aid in the weight loss battle or improve overall blood sugar control. If you use them, be careful not to exceed the acceptable daily intakes. Better still, use them only occasionally. If you insist upon daily use (for coffee, cereal, etc.), opt for sucralose (Splenda), which seems the least likely to be problematic in the long run.

TABLE 6.1 Nonnutritive Sweeteners

Saccharin (Sweet'N Low, Hermesetas)

Composition: Synthetic—synthesized from petroleum or coal and other chemicals

Sweetness vs. Sugar (Sucrose): 200-700 times sweeter than sugar

Properties: Heat stable with bitter aftertaste

Food Uses: U.S.—used in many foods and beverages, tabletop sweeteners, and chewing gum. Canada—available only as a tabletop sweetener and sold in tablet or powder form in pharmacies.

Acceptable Daily Intake (ADI): 5 mg/kg body weight

Cautions: Not recommended for use during pregnancy and lactation

Aspartame (Equal, Nutrasweet)

Composition: Two amino acids, aspartic acid and phenylalanine, joined by methanol

Sweetness vs. Sugar (Sucrose): 200 times sweeter than sugar

Properties: Not heat stable and no aftertaste

Food Uses: Used in tabletop sweeteners, cold breakfast cereal, gelatins, puddings, chewing gum, and carbonated beverages. Carbonated beverages account for 70% of its use.

Acceptable Daily Intake (ADI): 50 mg/kg body weight

Cautions: Should generally be avoided by those with pheylketonuria (PKU)

Acesulfame K (Sunett)

Composition: Synthetic—acesulfame plus potassium salt

Sweetness vs. Sugar (Sucrose): 200 times sweeter than sugar

Properties: Heat stable with a bitter aftertaste when used in large amounts

Food Uses: Used in tabletop sweeteners and as an additive in chewing gum, confections, desserts, yogurt, sauces, and alcoholic beverages

Acceptable Daily Intake (ADI): 15 mg/kg body weight

Cautions: May not be suitable for those on potassium-restricted diets or who have sulfa/antibiotic-based allergies

Sucralose (Splenda)

Composition: Trichlorinated sugar (3 hydrogen-oxygen groups in sucrose are replaced with 3 chlorine atoms)

Sweetness vs. Sugar (Sucrose): 600 times sweeter than sugar

Properties: Highly heat stable with no aftertaste

Food Uses: Used in tabletop sweeteners and in a number of desserts, confections, and nonalcoholic beverages. U.S.—not permitted.

Acceptable Daily Intake (ADI): 15 mg/kg body weight

Cautions: None

Cyclamate (Sucaryl, Sugar Twin, Weight Watchers)

Composition: Synthetic—sodium or calcium cyclamate

Sweetness vs. Sugar (Sucrose): 30 times sweeter than sugar

Properties: Heat stable with no aftertaste

Food Uses: U.S.—not permitted. Canada—available only as a tabletop sweetener and sold in tablet or powder form in pharmacies.

Acceptable Daily Intake (ADI): 11 mg/kg body weight

Cautions: Not recommended for use during pregnancy and lactation

STEVIA—A SWEET SOLUTION?

Stevia is an herb in the chrysanthemum family native to Paraguay that also grows in Brazil and Argentina and is widely cultivated in Asia. Stevia has been used for centuries to sweeten foods, including tea. Stevia leaves and herbal powder made from whole leaves are reported to be ten to fifteen times sweeter than table sugar. Refined extracts of stevia called steviosides (a white powder containing 85 to 95 percent steviosides) are approximately two to three hundred times sweeter than table sugar. Most stevia has a slightly bitter aftertaste and a faint herbal or licorice flavor. Stevioside powder is the nonnutritive sweetener of choice in Japan and is quickly gaining a stronghold in many Asian and South American countries. Regulatory agencies of these countries are convinced that the herb not only is safe for human consumption, but may offer potential health benefits. Clinical studies suggest that stevia may improve blood sugar control, protect liver function, fight infectious microorganisms, and have beneficial effects on fat absorption and blood pressure.

It all seems pretty straightforward until you review the status of stevia in the U.S. Since the mid-1980s, the FDA has absolutely refused to approve stevia for use as a noncaloric sweetener. Indeed, it has been labeled an "unsafe food additive," and a search-and-seizure campaign and full-fledged "import alert" have been issued against it. Although since 1994 stevia can be legally marketed as a dietary supplement, any reference to its use as a sweetener is strictly prohibited. Why? There are two schools of thought on this issue. The first is that there is not sufficient evidence supporting stevia's safety to approve it for widespread use. This is the view currently held by the FDA, Health Canada, and CSPI. Although there is no evidence of harm to people, some express concern that laboratory studies on animals suggest possible cancer and reproductive-health problems. The second school of thought declares that the FDA has been actively suppressing stevia for years, probably caving in to pressures from the politically powerful artificial sweeteners industry. Stevia would be a fearsome competitor—it is relatively cheap and it is natural—both features attractive to consumers. Who's right? While we don't know for sure, stevia has a long history of use, and the preponderance of evidence seems to support its safety, in our opinion. Dr. Andrew Weil, America's best known advocate for integrative medicine and director of the Program in Integrative Medicine at the University of Arizona, makes no apologies when he states that stevia is the best noncaloric sweetener available today. However, this is one question you may wish to do a little groundwork on yourself. The information on this topic is extensive and fascinating—definitely worth a look.

ALTERNATIVE NUTRITIVE SWEETENERS

Nutritive sweeteners are those that provide calories, including all sugars and sugar alcohols. However, not all sugars or sugar alcohols are created equal. They have varying nutritive values and differing impacts on blood sugar levels. For example, if glucose is the reference food with a glycemic index (GI) of 100, sucrose (table sugar) has a GI of 65, lactose (sugars found in milk) 46, and fructose (sugars found in fruit) 23. That means that fructose has only about one-third the glycemic effect of sucrose. In addition, fructose is about one and a half times sweeter than table sugar, which means you need less of it to produce a similar degree of sweetness. Sugar alcohols have minimal effects on blood sugar levels, although the foods that contain them are almost always carbohydrate-based, so those foods do affect blood sugar levels. The reason sucrose has a lower GI than glucose is because sucrose is half glucose and half fructose. Some sugars are 100 percent sucrose (table sugar), while others are different combinations of glucose, fructose, sucrose, and maltose. (Maltose is the sugar that makes up starch—when starch is broken down it is broken down into units of maltose. Maltose is two units of glucose.) It is important to note that consumption of large amounts of fructose (15 to 20 percent of daily calories) has been shown to increase total and LDL cholesterol in people with diabetes and total and LDL cholesterol and triglycerides in healthy individuals. So, while fructose does reduce glycemic response when compared to other sugars, it should be used in moderation.

Sugar Alcohols: Better Sugars for People with Diabetes?

Sugar alcohols, also known as polyols, include mannitol, sorbitol, xylitol, erythritol, isomalt, lactitol, maltitol, and hydrogenated starch hydrolysates (HSHs). They are found naturally in many plant foods, but are most concentrated in fruits and vegetables. Lactitol is derived from lactose, and HSHs from a mixture of sorbitol, maltitol, and hydrogenated oligosaccharides. Other sugar alcohols are derived from plant sources, including seaweeds.

Sugar alcohols are used as sweeteners and bulking agents in confections, ice cream, jams and jellies, fillings and frostings, beverages, baked products, and many so called "dietetic" foods that are labeled "sugar-free" or "no sugar added." People with diabetes often assume these foods are like "free foods" and will have little or no impact on the glycemic response. This is unfortunately not the case. While sugar alcohols produce a reduced glycemic response compared with similar amounts of sugar, they still have an effect on blood sugar. In addition, "dietetic" foods often contain other carbohydrates such as flour or rice, which impact blood sugar independently. Sometimes the "sugar-free" or "no added sugar" label simply serves as an excuse to overeat, resulting in even greater caloric intakes and glycemic responses than might occur with more moderate amounts of regular products.

Sugar alcohols have been designated by the FDA as "Generally Recognized as Safe," thus there is no requirement to designate an acceptable daily intake. The primary disadvantage of sugar alcohols is that, because they are incompletely absorbed in the intestine, they can have a laxative effect, especially when used in large quantity. For this reason, a declaration must appear on the label of any foods that, with reasonable ingestion, could result in the consumption of at least 20 grams of mannitol or 50 grams of sorbitol per day.

THE BOTTOM LINE

Sugar alcohols are safe in moderate amounts and have little impact on glycemic response. However, foods containing sugar alcohols are not "free foods," and many contain white flour or other concentrated carbohydrate sources, so they have a significant impact on blood sugars. Don't expect to save many calories buying special dietary products containing these sugars!

SUGAR OPTIONS—IS NATURAL BETTER?

While there is some truth to the old adage, "sugar is sugar is sugar," certain types of sugars do offer significant advantages over others. The balance of this chapter will explore some of the more popular unrefined or slightly refined sugars and consider their usefulness as sweeteners for people with diabetes. We'll look at dry sugars like raw sugar, Rapadura, Sucanat, and date sugar, as well as liquid sugars like agave syrup, blackstrap molasses, barley malt, brown rice syrup, maple syrup, and honey.

Refined Sugars
Refined sugars include all those sugars that are extracted from plants and are purified to yield sugar. Table sugar is made from sugar cane or sugar beets. Glucose, often seen in processed foods, comes from high-starch foods such as corn. Fructose (also called levulose) is extracted from sugar, which is 50 percent fructose. (While fruits are a great source of fructose, it would be way too expensive to extract fructose from these foods.) Prior to refining, the plants used to derive these sugars contain a number of vitamins and minerals; however, after refining almost all of these nutrients are gone, leaving only pure sucrose, glucose, or fructose. Brown sugar is produced using a combination of white sugar and molasses, and contains some minerals, depending upon the amount of molasses present. While brown sugar does contribute some minerals, the contribution to overall nutrient intake is insignificant.

Raw, Unrefined, or Lightly Refined Sweeteners
Raw, unrefined, or lightly refined sweeteners offer several advantages over their more refined counterparts. First, they generally contain some nutrients, although considering the small quantities consumed, the contribution is generally insignificant. (There are some exceptions.) Second, some less-refined sugars have a lower glycemic index than sucrose, although this is not always the case. Table 6.2 provides a description of the various less-refined sugar alternatives.

THE BOTTOM LINE

Sugars, refined or otherwise, should not be used in excess as they can crowd out more nutritious foods and adversely affect glycemic control. Some unrefined sugars offer benefits in terms of nutritional value and/or glycemic response. The one caloric sweetener that stands out above all the others for people with blood sugar challenges is agave syrup, which has a lower glycemic index than any other nutritive sweetener. Remember that agave syrup is mainly fructose, which can adversely affect blood lipids when used in excess.

TABLE 6.2 Nutritive Sweeteners

Raw sugar

Coarse, minimally refined sugar made from sugar cane or sugar beets.

Several minerals retained, most vitamins lost. Glycemic response similar to sucrose.

1 cup (250 mL) replaces 1 cup of sugar in recipes.

Turbinado sugar

A coarse sugar, slightly more refined than raw sugar—made from sugar cane or sugar beets.

Contains small amounts of minerals (slightly greater than brown sugar). Glycemic response similar to sucrose.

1 cup (250 mL) replaces 1 cup of sugar in recipes.

Sucanat

Once made from freshly squeezed cane juice (until the company changed ownership and the processing technique). Today Sucanat is still considered a "granulated cane juice," but is made by mixing refined cane juice and molasses.

Contains some minerals (per 100 g of product: 60 mg potassium, 148 mg calcium, and 4 mg of iron). Glycemic response similar to sucrose.

1 cup (250 mL) replaces 1 cup of sugar in recipes.

Rapadura

Granulated sugar from evaporated cane juice, freshly squeezed from sugar cane.

Most nutrient dense of cane sugars (per 100 g of product: 600-1,000 mg potassium, 80-110 calcium, and 40-100 mg magnesium). May provide a slightly lower glycemic response compared with sucrose. Mild caramel flavor.

1 cup (250 mL) replaces 1 cup of sugar in recipes.

Date sugar

Made from ground, dehydrated dates.

Has the same nutrients as dates. However, when used as a sugar, overall contribution to nutrient intake is small. Doesn't dissolve when added to liquids. Very expensive.

1 cup (250 mL) replaces 1 cup of sugar in some recipes.

Agave syrup

Extracted from the blue agave plant native to Mexico.

Some vitamins and minerals. Is 90% fructose, so has an exceptionally low glycemic index. The glycemic index of agave syrup has been reported to been extremely low (10-11) for syrups with a fructose content of approximately 90%, and higher (39) for syrups with a fructose content of 57-71%

½ cup (125 mL) syrup replaces 1 cup (250 mL) of sugar in recipes
(reduce liquid by ¼ cup/60mL).

Blackstrap molasses

A by-product of sugar refining remaining after the final extraction of the sugar.

The only sugar with significant nutritional value, even when consumed in moderate amounts. Two tablespoons of blackstrap molasses (30 mL) provides about 7.2 mg of iron and 352 mg of calcium. Can contain residues from chemicals used in growing and refining the sugar cane or sugar beet (organic options are available).

Does not replace sugar well. Small amounts can replace liquid sweeteners.

Barley malt

Made from soaked, sprouted whole barley. The sprouts are dried, mixed with water, and cooked until a syrup is produced.

Small amounts of vitamins and minerals. Glycemic index similar to sucrose. Only 40% as sweet as sugar. Rich malt flavor.

Use 1⅓ cups (333 mL) to replace 1 cup of sugar (reduce liquid by ¼ cup/60 mL).

Brown rice syrup

Made from brown rice, water, and a natural cereal enzyme to break down the starches to sugar.

Small amounts of vitamins and minerals. Glycemic index similar to sucrose. About half as sweet as sugar.

Does not replace sugar well. Can be used to replace honey.

Maple syrup

From the sap of maple trees.

Trace amounts of vitamins and minerals. 90-100% sucrose, therefore has a similar glycemic index.

Use ⅔ cup (165 mL) to replace 1 cup of sugar (reduce liquid by ¼ cup/60 mL)

Honey

Refined by bees. Bees collect nectar and change it in their stomach into glucose and fructose, which is eventually regurgitated into the honeycomb.

Contains small amounts of vitamins and minerals. Glycemic index of about 73 (slightly higher than sucrose because sucrose is half fructose and honey is about 40% fructose). 20-60% sweeter than sugar.

Use ⅔ cup (165 mL) to replace 1 cup (250 mL) of sugar (reduce liquid by ¼ cup/60 mL)

CHAPTER 7

Defensive Dining

J ust when this new, healthful eating style becomes second nature, the universe throws you a curve ball—Christmas holidays, summer vacation, a big birthday bash, or a night on the town. Special occasions such as these seem to grow more elaborate and drawn out with each passing year. Christmas seems to begin the moment the last morsel of Thanksgiving pumpkin pie is swallowed. Boxes of chocolates, bowls of candy, and trays of cookies and fruitcake begin to appear in the office. Then come the staff parties, open houses, and family festivities—each event being more food-centered than the next. How can anyone survive such consistent temptation unscathed?

Your most powerful defense is to be prepared! This chapter will help you respond to challenges in a way that fully supports health and healing. This doesn't mean you'll learn the fine art of how to deprive yourself or avoid celebrations—quite the contrary! A truly healthy response is one that recognizes the immense value of special times with friends and family and embraces them with love and laughter. The key is to reinvent traditions and celebrations, keeping the best of the old and recreating new, more healthful traditions that better support our well-being.

Defensive Dining

Whether it is dinner at a fancy restaurant, a quick fast-food stop on your way home from work, or a treat at the movies, the very thought of eating out can be stressful for people with diabetes. Fortunately, with a little know-how, you can once again look forward to wonderful dining adventures. Today, healthful options are more popular than ever, and almost all eating establishments provide a least a few decent choices.

The primary concerns about eating out generally fall into one of five categories.

✓ Choice of restaurant
✓ Calories
✓ Fat
✓ Refined carbohydrates
✓ Timing

CHOOSING A RESTAURANT

Ethnic restaurants are generally a good bet, especially if the traditional cuisine is plant-based, as is the case for Asian, Mediterranean, Middle Eastern, Mexican, Indian, and South American restaurants. Vegetarian and vegan restaurants offer some wonderfully unique and nutritious options. In many larger cities there are excellent gourmet vegetarian restaurants that serve truly world-class foods. North American family-style restaurants generally offer at least two or three decent selections, such as stir-fries with rice, veggie burgers with salad, and pasta with vegetable-based sauces. North American or European fine dining restaurants usually have fairly limited options; however, if you call ahead, the chef may be willing to prepare something quite extraordinary. If you are going for fast food, look for a place that offers salads, veggie burgers, baked potatoes, or bean burritos.

Calorie-Saving Tips

When you are trying to limit calories (1,400 to 1,800 calories on most weight loss diets), you need to have to have some idea of the energy content of various popular menu items. Table 7.1 provides the calorie and fat content of a selection of restaurant favorites. You can see that not only is it a challenge to stay within your allotted calories for any given meal, but you can easily exceed your entire day's intake in a single meal if you aren't careful. For example, an order of potato skins and a large cola would set you back almost 1,500 calories! The following calorie-savings tips will help you keep calories within your limits.

✓ Avoid "supersized" portions—this is simply a consumer-friendly way of saying "super stacked with calories." Items described as jumbo, deluxe, man-sized, hungry man, or extralarge are not much better. They are marketed as a bargain because of portion size, but they are no bargain for your waistline or your health.

✓ Order half portions—many restaurants offer half portions, and the servings are often quite generous. If you are having an appetizer or a dessert, this is definitely the way to go.

✓ If you are a senior, take advantage of senior portions—these meals are both more reasonably sized and more economical.

✓ Share with your dining partner, especially when you know servings are generous. This instantly cuts your calories in half. A typical serving of pasta at an Italian restaurant is three to four cups. Cutting this in half would still give you a very generous serving!

✓ Avoid desserts—some restaurant desserts have more calories than the entrée. If you do order dessert, go for fresh or baked fruit or sherbet. If you opt for something more decadent, be sure to share it with at least one other person.

✓ Ask for a take-home container—decide ahead of time how much is reasonable to eat. For example, if you order a small pizza containing 700 calories, eating only two-thirds of the pizza will bring it down to 462 calories.

✓ Ask for substitutions—don't be afraid to ask to switch meal items. For example, replace fries with a salad and ask for the dressing on the side. This one change will save you about 200 calories.

✓ Limit fillers—buns, bread, tortilla chips, and other freebies that come with your meal can put you over the top before your meal even arrives. Two large slices of Italian bread with butter or olive oil and balsamic vinegar has about 350 calories, and 2 ounces of tortilla chips (twenty chips) with salsa has about 300 calories.

✓ Steer clear of buffets—they are notorious triggers for overeating. Some restaurants offer soup and salad bars with regular meals. If you go for a soup and salad bar, skip the regular meal! Load your plate with fresh vegetables, and go lightly on the creamy, mayonnaise-based salads. Keep your portions of salad dressing small or opt for reduced-calorie dressings.

Keeping a Lid on the Fat

Fat is two and a half times more concentrated in calories than carbohydrates or protein. Just one tablespoon of fat adds 100 calories to what you are eating without increasing the quantity of food. Even though fat does not directly raise blood sugar levels, excess fat contributes to obesity, insulin resistance, heart disease, and hypertension.

✓ Avoid anything deep-fried—these foods are literally swimming in artery-clogging fat, the type that is either high in saturated fats or trans fatty acids. Most battered foods are deep-fried.

✓ Ask if the chef can go lightly on added fats in preparing your meal. For example, ask if the bare minimum amount of oil can be used in preparing your stir-fry.

✓ Request high-fat toppings be omitted or served "on the side." Salad dressings, butter, sour cream, grated cheese, gravy, and similar optional toppings are high in fat and cause calories to quickly escalate. For example, a salad containing 50 calories would increase to 90 calories with the addition of one to two tablespoons of reduced-calorie dressing. However, if you top your salad with cheese, croutons, bacon bits, and a creamy dressing, the calorie count jumps to about 500 calories.

✓ If you order soup, select one that is broth-based instead of cream-based. Cream soups can easily contain 400 calories and over 25 grams of fat, while broth-based soups are generally low in fat and about half the calories.

✓ Select tomato- or other vegetable-based sauces rather than cream sauces.

✓ Ask for low-fat milk or even skim milk rather than cream for your coffee, tea, or cereal.

✓ If you are ordering meat, opt for fish—preferably broiled, baked, or poached.

✓ Choose raw, grilled, or steamed vegetables over marinated or creamed vegetables.

✓ If you know the fat content of a restaurant meal is going to be on the high side, offset the extra fat in the meal by cutting back on the fat the rest of the day.

✓ If you go for the bread, skip the butter.

✓ If you opt for higher-fat menu items, order the smallest size available, share with your dining partner, or bring half home in a doggie bag.

Reducing Refined Carbohydrates

Refined carbohydrates are staples in our culture, so it comes as no surprise that they are difficult to avoid. Unfortunately, selecting meatless options does not necessarily solve the problem. The most popular meatless meals in North American restaurants are pasta, pizza, and veggie burgers—all of which generally feature refined grains. So how does one minimize intake of refined carbohydrates when opting for meatless meals? Consider the following suggestions.

✓ Look for vegetarian and vegan restaurants. These are probably the easiest places to find whole grains like quinoa, barley, wheat berries, brown rice, and whole grain breads.

✓ Go ethnic. Many ethnic restaurants focus on vegetables, legumes, and rice. While white rice is the usual accompaniment, some do offer brown rice, so be sure to ask.

✓ If ordering pasta, choose one with a tomato- or vegetable-based sauce, and don't eat all of it, as restaurant portions are usually far larger than a reasonable portion for a person watching calories and carbohydrates.

✓ Include a big salad or a cup of bean soup with your meal for extra fiber.

✓ Go for whole grain breads if you have the option. If only white breads are served, let the management know you'd appreciate whole grain breads. (Every request helps!)

✓ Forgo dessert—most are not only white flour–based, but also loaded with sugar.

✓ Be innovative with snack choices when eating out—many popular snacks such as pretzels, muffins, bagels, cookies, and other baked goods are white flour–based. Instead, order a fresh fruit smoothie or some low-fat popcorn.

Timing

If you do not take insulin and/or sulfonylureas, careful timing of meals is not as critical, although having some consistency of meal timing is a good practice. The main concern about delaying a meal when you are on insulin and/or

TABLE *7.1* Energy and Fat Content of Selected Restaurant Favorites

Type of Food	Calories	Fat Grams
Appetizers		
Hot and sour soup, 8 oz. (250 mL)	60	3
Buffalo wings, 12 wings, 13 oz. (369 g)	700	48
Fried mozzarella sticks, 9 sticks, 8 oz. (227 g)	830	51
Stuffed potato skins, 8 skins, 12 oz. (340 g)	1,120	79
Main Dishes		
Chili, large, 12 oz. (340 g)	310	10
Veggie sub, 12-inch (no mayo or cheese)	400	6
Chicken breast fillet sandwich, 1	430	16
Vegetarian pizza, 2 slices	480	18
Deluxe double burger, 1	540	30
Pepperoni pizza, 2 slices	700	34
Deluxe pizza, personal pan	720	34
Beef burrito, 14 oz. (398 g)	830	40
Moussaka (ground beef/eggplant dish), 12 oz. (340 g)	830	48
Chicken fajitas, 2 cups (500 mL), 4 small tortillas	840	24
Tuna sub, 12-inch (no mayo or cheese)	880	46
Turkey pot pie	910	45
Lasagne, 2 cups, 20 oz. (500 mL, 568 g)	960	53
Chicken strip basket (with fries)	1,000	50
Meatball Classic Sub, Subway, 12-inch (no mayo or cheese)	1,020	52
Taco salad, 3½ cups (875 mL)	1,100	71
Fettuccine alfredo, 2½ cups (625 mL)	1,500	97
Kung pao chicken with rice, 4½ cups (1,125 mL)	1,620	76
Side Dishes		
Mixed vegetables, 5 oz. (142 g)	130	9
Fried rice, 8 oz. (227 g)	430	13
Hot stuffed baked potato, broccoli and cheese, 14 oz. (398 g)	470	14
French fries, fast food, large	520	24
Loaded baked potato (bacon, butter, cheese, sour cream), 1 medium	620	31
New York fries, regular, 10 oz. (284 g)	860	48
Onion rings, 11	900	64

Type of Food	Calories	Fat Grams
Beverages		
Diet cola, 16 oz. (454 mL)	0	0
Cappuccino, 16 oz. (454 mL)	120	3
Cola, small, 12 oz. (340 mL)	155	0
Fruit smoothie, 16 oz. (454 mL)	160	1
Caffé latte with skim milk, 16 oz. (454 mL)	160	1
Orange juice, 16 oz. (454 mL)	197	0
Ice tea, sweetened, 19 oz. (539 mL)	200	0
Lemonade, 15 oz. (426 mL)	240	0
Slush, medium, 32 oz. (905 mL)	290	0
Cola, large, 26 oz. (770 mL)	336	0
Café mocha with whole milk and whipped cream, 16 oz. (474 mL)	420	23
Caramel corretto, 16 oz. (454 g)	440	9
Chocolate milkshake, 19 oz. (540 mL)	720	18
Chocolate malt, 20 oz. (568 mL)	880	22
Desserts/Snacks		
Orange fruit juice bar, 1	60	0
Yogurt cone, 8 oz. (228 g)	267	6
Low-fat carrot muffin, 4½ oz. (128 g)	280	2
Cookie, milk chocolate with walnuts, 1 large, 2½ oz. (71 g)	320	17
Black Forest cake, ⅛ of cake	320	13
Pretzel, soft, 1 with topping	340	5
Apple fritter, 3½ oz. (100 g)	340	15
Chocolate chip muffin, 4½ oz. (128 g)	430	16
Frosted fudge brownie, 4 oz. (114 g)	440	21
Apple cinnamon Danish, 4 oz. (114 g)	440	20
Carrot muffin, regular, 4½ oz. (128 g)	450	19
Apple pie, 4 oz. piece (114 g)	490	22
Dipped cone, medium (220 g)	490	24
Classic chocolate ice cream, 2 scoops	520	28
Classic French vanilla ice cream, 2 scoops	570	36
Cinnamon bun, 7 oz. (199 g)	720	27
Cookie Dough Blizzard (439 g)	950	36
Fudge brownie sundae, 10 oz. (284 g)	1,130	57

sulfonylureas is that your blood sugar could dip too low and you could become hypoglycemic. There are several reasonable ways of dealing with meal delays so you can avoid hypoglycemic reactions. It is best, however, to discuss the possibilities with your health care team, so they can help to determine what will work best for you. For those taking insulin or oral medications, see pages 171-72 in chapter 10.

SPECIAL OCCASIONS

Holidays and special occasions provide us with great joy, incredible connections, cherished memories, and a whole lot of stress. For people with diabetes, the stress often takes center stage. You may be concerned about how to provide the kind of food people expect and still maintain any sort of diet yourself. You may be thoroughly convinced that simply looking at the triple-fudge layer cake will add ten pounds to your waistline. Rather than consuming yourself with worry, plan your defense! Here are five simple steps to start you on the right track.

Five Steps to Healthful, Happy Celebrations

1. Serve nutritious fare. So often, we assume that people want the most decadent food available. The truth is, many people feel constantly overstuffed during festive occasions. Many try very hard to set in place a sort of damage control for festive times. So, when you are the person doing the entertaining, surprise your guests with a healthful gourmet feast. Most will be absolutely delighted with the lighter cuisine. For appetizers, serve bruschetta, stuffed grape leaves, sushi rolls, lettuce wraps, crackers and antipasto, pickled asparagus, artichoke hearts, and raw veggies with a light dip. For your main course, consider going for plant-based ethnic main dishes. Asian themes are especially interesting and enjoyable. For dessert, how about a fruit salad with some thin, crispy cookies or a pudding layered with raspberry sauce? Enjoy!

2. Bring wholesome offerings when you are invited out. Whether it's a staff party, a potluck dinner, or a house party, make your contribution stand out as being both nutritious and delicious. If you are invited for a small dinner party, offer to make a significant contribution to the meal.

3. Increase your activity during the holidays. This will help compensate for the natural increase in food consumption, help with managing your hunger, and make you feel a whole lot better.

4. Don't skip meals. It is so tempting to skip a meal or two when you know that there is going to be a big meal at night. Resist the temptation. Skipping meals is risky for those on medication and not a healthful choice for anyone. When you skip breakfast or lunch (or both), you set yourself up for a night-time binge.

5. Enjoy your favorites in moderation. While you don't have to pass up all your favorite treats, it is important to be selective and eat moderate serving sizes. For example, if you absolutely love shortbread cookies, forgo the butter tarts, fruitcake, and chocolate fudge and allow yourself a couple of cookies. Savor them with a cup of tea. At dinner, enjoy small servings of rich foods like stuffing and mashed potatoes, but pile on the vegetables. Remember that serving sizes make a huge difference to your final calorie count. For example, a large slice of carrot cake ($\frac{1}{8}$ of an 8- or 9-inch cake) will set you back about 520 calories while a small piece of carrot cake ($\frac{1}{16}$ of that cake) will cost only 260 calories.

TRAVEL

If you think that diabetes makes it too difficult to travel, you are in for a pleasant surprise. Even people who rely on insulin injections can enjoy vacations around the world. For individuals who control their diabetes with diet and exercise alone, travel is a snap. For those on insulin, more preparation is required; however, the dividends pay off in a safe and rewarding trip.

About a month before your trip, visit your doctor for a checkup. It is important that your diabetes is under good control prior to your departure. If you take insulin and are flying or leaving the country, you'll need a letter from your doctor describing your medical condition and outlining the medical supplies you require. If you are getting any vaccinations, be sure to get them several weeks before you leave, as they can sometimes adversely affect diabetes control. Your health care team will also need to help you adjust your insulin or medications if you are crossing time zones.

There are several items you will need to bring with you. First, be sure to carry or wear appropriate diabetes identification. This can be a bracelet or an identification card. As you know, when hypoglycemia strikes, your brain ceases to function normally and these items can save your life! Proper identification gives others the information that you may not be able to give in an emergency. You will also need to bring an extra supply of insulin, syringes, medications, and test strips, especially if you are traveling to another country.

You never know when you might be delayed by a week or more. If you take insulin, you'll need to buy a special insulated bag to ensure it does not freeze or get too hot. Finally, take along some comfortable walking shoes. They should be well broken in before your trip.

Travel by Air

Airlines are well experienced in accommodating passengers with diabetes. It is important to notify them ahead of time and order a special meal. Regardless of whether or not meals are served, it is important to bring along extra snacks if you are on insulin or sulfonylureas, just in case of meal delays. You'll also need to drink plenty of fluids, preferably water.

Be sure to always carry your medical supplies with you on the plane. *Never* pack them in your luggage, as there is always a chance that the luggage could be delayed or lost.

Travel by Car/Bus/Train

Once again, you'll need to pack along some food, especially if you are on insulin or sulfonylureas. Bring handy snacks such as dried or fresh fruit and granola or energy bars, and perhaps even a sandwich in case you miss a meal. Stick to your usual meal and snack times as much as possible, and drink plenty of fluids. Be sure to keep the food in carry-on luggage if traveling by bus or train. Take full advantage of every break to get a little exercise in— even a short walk can be helpful.

You've Arrived!

If you are on insulin, store it in a cool place as soon as you can. Get oriented. Check out where the nearest medical clinic, hospital, and pharmacy are located.

Check your blood sugar frequently, as your routine is often quite different than it is at home. If you are walking a lot, be sure to check your feet for blisters. Avoid walking barefoot on the beach.

If you are traveling with a friend or staying with someone, be sure to let him or her know how to recognize a hypoglycemic reaction and how to effectively treat it.

Enjoy your vacation!

CHAPTER 8

The Essentials of Living Well

N ow that you have your food choices down to a fine art, it is time to turn our attention to other vital aspects of lifestyle. This chapter will walk you through the essentials of living well: physical fitness, sleep, sexual fitness, and emotional health.

PHYSICAL WELLNESS

If you could bottle the benefits of exercise and put them into a pill, the line of people to buy that magic potion would be endless. When you look at the people best equipped to handle the hurdles of life, the fittest have the most resilience.

Not only do we need the best food for our bodies to function, our bodies need to be efficient processors of that fuel. We are all built to be vigorous creatures and yet we (and subsequently our children) are less active than we were only a few decades ago. We need to change that. While a sedentary lifestyle remains one of the biggest factors leading to heart attack and stroke, it's also a major contributor to obesity and diabetes. Diet alone cannot remedy the effects of inactivity.

In a recent edition of the prestigious *New England Journal of Medicine,* the editorial board of the *Journal* stated that those of us who are in shape live the longest. In addition, it would take just three to six months for a regular fitness program to show measurable results in terms of fitness and health benefits. The benefits this study measured exceed what is strictly measurable, like cholesterol levels and glucose tolerance, the reduction of obesity, and the lowering of blood pressure. There are also positive effects on the tone and reactivity of blood vessels, on the balance of the nervous system, on the "stickiness" of the blood, and on overall inflammation, and all of these appear to be significant factors in modifying cardiovascular risk, and ultimately in increasing survival.

All of the major medical organizations concur that everyone needs to adopt a physically active lifestyle, and all adults should incorporate at least thirty minutes of moderately intense physical activity on most or preferably all days of the week. The prestigious National Research Council has recommended a goal of an hour of exercise a day as optimal: this is the most ambitious recommendation for fitness that we have yet seen.

It appears we can live longer simply by living well. What is more, it is not only the length of our lives that improves with fitness, but the quality of living. When we are active and vigorous, our strength and stamina for daily living remain at or near their peak, despite the passage of time. Our balance is better and our mood improves. It has been shown that the most effective treatment for mild to moderate depression is vigorous exercise. It is more beneficial than medication or counseling, and the effects are longer lasting. On the other hand, exercise is a perfect complement to both medications and a counseling program. In fact, it may be that the insights gained in a relationship with a trusted counselor or advisor are processed more fully during exercise.

All of our vital organs function better when our bodies are fit. With good blood circulation, the brain can more quickly respond to imbalances throughout the body, fine-tuning the need for hormonal regulation of insulin, growth hormone, estrogen, testosterone, or adrenaline. All of the cellular needs for nutritional support or waste removal are easily met. When our immune system gets regular stimulation, we are less likely to get ill, catch a cold or flu, or even contract cancer.

DEVELOPING THE EXERCISE HABIT

If you find it difficult to take up exercise, remember the words of a famous Japanese martial arts instructor: "You can't help how you feel, but you can help what you do!" Building a varied fitness program into your lifestyle will bring in untold benefits for even the smallest effort.

A vigorous, active lifestyle is best achieved with an approach that balances cardiovascular fitness, such as running or walking, with muscular development and agility. Large studies have shown that a lifestyle that included twenty minutes of vigorous activity three times a week was more effective in lengthening lives than one where cholesterol levels were reduced without incorporating exercise.

What are the elements of our "Live Well" exercise program for defeating diabetes? Like eating well, these principles are adapted to any individual's personal perspective, but represent choices from three main areas.

1. Cardiovascular fitness (aerobic exercise)
2. Strength training
3. Flexibility

Cardiovascular Fitness

Aerobic exercise improves stamina and fitness levels, and gives us the energy to be fit and active. Especially in terms of extending lifespan, aerobic fitness and cardiovascular workouts pay off with big rewards. But even in terms of daily living, extra cardiac and lung reserves are a big plus. Any little cold or flu, or even bronchitis or pneumonia, can be less of a threat because we have the extra metabolic efficiency that allows us to overcome our impairment from an illness.

The best results from cardiovascular fitness would result from workouts totaling sixty minutes a day. As our capacity for vigorous activity develops, this exercise could be more and more intense. Weight-bearing exercise is best; brisk walking (at least four miles per hour), jogging, cross-country skiing, snow-shoeing, roller blading, playing soccer or basketball, racquetball, and squash are all great choices. Chopping wood and carrying water can also qualify if you keep up a steady pace, and so can working up the garden in spring and fall, weeding vigorously; even raking and hoeing are all helpful.

While at one time experts believed that exercise had to be continuous for at least 15 to 20 minutes to count as an aerobic workout, we have since learned that cumulative exercise counts. Running up the stairs at work, walking from the far corners of the parking lot, riding a bicycle to work, and all other short bursts of activity are great additions to a daily workout.

If possible, do your aerobic activities with friends, in a fitness class, or on a team, as the energy of group is often a great motivator. Family sporting activity, like badminton, tennis, racquet ball, and trampolining, can be great for fitness. Bicycling in groups can be both vigorous and wonderfully aerobic, but wear helmets and use bicycle paths rather than streets whenever possible.

Equipment-aided workouts can be easy on the joints if the machinery is properly set up. Elliptical trainers, cross-country ski machines, treadmills with inclines and arm poles, stationary and reclining bicycles, rowing machines, and step climbers are excellent and relatively easy on the knees. Any of these activities can be closely approximated by simply running up and down the stairs, of course, but the main issue is both enjoyment and safety.

When it comes to aerobic activity, the big challenge for most people is finding something they like and sticking to it. If you are going to succeed in making aerobic activity a part of your daily routine, it must become a priority—something that doesn't get tossed aside unless you are in bed with the flu. Additionally, it must become part of your usual routine, like eating and sleeping. That means you need to ask yourself when it would best fit into your day. Are you a morning person or a night owl? If you are a morning person, consider fitting your exercise in first thing after you wake up. If you are a night owl, evening classes may work best. If you are going to stick with it for the long haul, you must pick activities you enjoy. It's best if you include a variety of different things. For example, in the summer you may opt for swimming, biking, and baseball, while in the winter you may prefer to play indoor tennis during the week and go cross-country skiing on the weekends. Think back to when you were a teenager or young adult. What did you really enjoy? If you were a swimmer, consider a masters swim club. If you were a badminton player, join a local league. If you weren't athletic at all, think about what you always wished you could do. Do it. Take lessons. Don't worry about what anyone thinks. Just have fun.

Depending on your age, it is sensible to work up to your capacity for vigorous aerobic exercise gradually. If you're over the age of forty (or younger if you have a family history of early heart disease), then consider a cardiac stress test using monitored exercise to determine how much activity your heart can handle. These exercise stress tests are also recommended whenever any unexplained symptoms develop.

Measuring Your Aerobic Fitness

One of the simplest measures of fitness is resting heart rate. People who exercise regularly have low resting heart rates; sedentary people have higher resting heart rates. A large Italian study showed that people with a more rapid heart rate were over 50 percent more likely to die from all causes, not just cardiovascular disease. Heart rate is a simple measure of fitness, and we can change our heart rate to lower, more beneficial levels just by regularly exercising.

To get an idea of your maximum suggested heart rate with exercise, simply subtract your age from 220 beats per minute (bpm). If you are forty years old, your maximum suggested heart rate would be 220 minus 40, or 180 bpm.

Maximum Heart Rate = 220 – Age in Years

Aim for 70 to 85 percent of your maximum rate as a goal, and try to sustain that for around twenty minutes a session.

Again, if you're forty, set your upper and lower desirable heart rates for working out by taking 70 percent of 180 bpm, which would be 126 bpm, and 85 percent of 180, which would be 153 bpm. You would want to exercise at a heart rate between 126 and 153 bpm for at least twenty minutes. If you were able to do this at least three times a week, you would get the benefits that accrue from overall aerobic fitness.

The nice thing about using a target heart rate range is that it automatically takes into account your fitness level. As you become more fit, you will have to exercise more vigorously to maintain the higher heart rate, because it will take more effort for you to increase your heart rate to reach your goal. This encourages more activity and results in an increase in your level of fitness, automatically!

Age	Target Heart Rate (range)
25-29	134-166
30-34	130-162
35-39	127-157
40-44	123-153
45-49	120-149
50-54	116-145
55-59	112-140
60-64	109-136
65-69	106-132
70-74	102-128
75-79	99-123
80-84	95-119
85-89	92-115

Strength Training

Strength or resistance training promotes muscular development, enhances lean body mass, boosts bone density, and provides the motor power to help us maintain a high degree of independence in our daily lives. With adequate muscle strength we can accomplish so much more in our day-to-day lives with ease. Our capacity for work increases and, especially as we age, the differences in our ability to perform tasks that require strength will be greatly enhanced. In one Boston study, the addition of strength training with light weights of one to five pounds for several short sessions each week increased the ability of people in their eighties and nineties to carry out the activities of daily living by as much as 300 percent. While we might not see such dramatic results, most of us would benefit from an increase in muscle mass.

Again, the good news is that with even a minimal workout, a remarkable increase in personal capacity results. For most people, resistance training means using weights. However, if you prefer to do pull-ups, push-ups, dips, or other resistance exercises using your own body weight, you'll find them just as effective. If you are going to the local community center or fitness club, you can easily alternate every other day between aerobic and strength workouts. If you prefer to do daily aerobics, you could include a short weight-training session that alternates various muscle groups. Also, have a few small weight sets around your home or at work that you can use when you take a break. It will make TV watching or sitting at the computer enlivening and physically profitable. These tips will help to optimize the effectiveness of your weight-training program.

✓ If possible, work with a qualified trainer who will tailor your program to suit your goals, abilities, and time, and monitor your progress.

✓ Allow sufficient recovery time after weight training. Two to three times a week is sufficient for most people—more is not better! Train on alternate days—do not work the same muscle groups two days in a row.

✓ Free weights are very effective and less expensive than renting or purchasing weight machines. You can use a combination of machines and free weights or stick to free weights exclusively.

✓ Use multiple series or "sets" of repetitions (two to four sets with eight to twelve repetitions per set) for big muscle gains. Decrease the number of repetitions while you increase weights as you progress.

✓ Use weights that are challenging. Go light with you first set (50 percent of maximum), heavier on your second (about 75 percent of maximum), and all out on your third (95 to 100 percent of maximum).

✓ Change exercises and weight about every four to six weeks. By challenging different muscles, you avoid getting into a rut that will slow down your progress.

Flexibility

Finally, along with aerobics and strength training, you'll need to incorporate a flexibility program into your routine. Flexibility is another key component of overall physical fitness. It is sometimes referred to as range of motion, the movement around your joints and the connecting muscles, tendons, ligaments, and bones.

For many people, flexibility begins to decline in their late twenties or early thirties, and continues to decline with increasing age. The best way to maintain flexibility is to work at it consistently and increase your stretching time as you get older. Muscle tightness and joint stiffness are natural consequences of inactivity. Frequent stretching helps reduce muscle tension, improve circulation, prevent injuries, and increase range of motion. Stretching after exercise also helps to prevent soreness.

Daily stretching is definitely the best way to enjoy major improvements. Periodic, hard stretching sessions often end up in injury and don't do much to improve your overall flexibility in the long run. Like aerobic exercise and strength training, stretching should involve gradual but significant challenges for maximum improvement. A good stretching program will put a lot of emphasis on proper mechanics and alignment, in order to reduce risk of injury. Static stretching (going into a position and holding it for at least ten seconds) is among the most effective methods of reducing muscle soreness and increasing flexibility. In addition, this type of stretching rarely results in injury.

It is important to stretch before and after aerobic activity, with lighter stretching prior to your workout and more intense stretching after the activity, when you are well warmed up. Before you stretch, get your muscles warm! If you are new to exercise, you will need to do light exercise for at least five minutes before stretching.

Certainly, any stretching regimen will help, but the practice of yoga has been especially rewarding for many people. Incorporating even simple breathing techniques and stimulating exercises adds a useful dimension that enhances fitness at many levels. Hatha yoga training (involving stretching and flexibility) and its cousins tai chi and qi gong have been in use for centuries. Tai chi and chi gong feature different series of movements that slowly flow from one position to another, like a dance in slow motion. Choosing one or the other of these ancient practices is a personal choice and often depends on the availability of a teacher or local class. Find a qualified instructor or personal trainer that you can trust; even some popular video or audio instruction tape sets would be a great start.

SLEEPING FOR FITNESS

In our hurry-up lives, we are rather like the White Rabbit in Alice in Wonderland running around reciting, "I'm late, I'm late, for a very important date; no time to say hello, goodbye, I'm late, I'm late!" Is it any wonder that many of us have neither the time for enough sleep nor the ability to achieve restful, restorative sleep when we do have the time?

When we incorporate fitness into the fabric of our day, we counteract the stress hormones that are generated by the fast pace of our lives. We prepare ourselves naturally for a peaceful, restful sleep by literally burning away the anxiety of a stress-filled day. With exercise, we can replace the hormones cortisol and adrenaline that our bodies use to meet the demands of a busy day with natural anxiety- and pain-relieving hormones: endorphins.

Preparing Yourself for a Good Night's Rest

Sleep does take some effort. Like any other aspect of a healthy and supportive lifestyle, sleep requires some level of conscious preparation. We need to understand that watching an eventful evening news program followed by two espresso coffees may not be the best preparation for a period of rest. Instead, if we have a warm bath with some Epsom salts dissolved in the water, we would relax our muscles and produce more serotonin (which enhances relaxation and relieves anxiety) and melatonin (which promotes sleep).

Current research suggests that the hours of sleep we get before midnight are the most restorative, but our setting is also very important. With the flood lights of neighbors' houses often shining into our bedrooms, or the street lights brightening up our entire houses all night long, light pollution is an increasing problem for this society. Recent findings suggest this is most harmful to the successful production of melatonin. Even a little light coming in under a door apparently prevents adequate relaxation and true rest. Although it may not be entirely easy, it would be best to choose a quiet, very dark setting in which to sleep at night. As well, wearing an eye mask is often helpful, and it's an inexpensive solution that is well tolerated and easy to obtain. Some people also benefit from eye pillows. These are not only a mask but also have a little filling in them which puts gentle weight on the eyes and helps with relaxation of the eye muscles.

A hot bath, followed by a few long, slow, deep breaths in and out, can help promote a restful night of sleep. Take the time for a brief relaxation with meditation or a prayer, and bring the mind to a place of inspired yet restful acceptance, a place of freedom from fears and the pressing burdens of personal responsibilities. A clean, uncluttered bedroom also helps prepare the mind for sleep.

Sleep Disorders

If others say you snore, if you are waking yourself up with loud breathing or loud snorts, or you feel like you are choking during the night, consider attending a sleep laboratory to see if you have sleep apnea. Sleep apnea is literally the inability to breathe properly while sleeping. It is caused when relaxation of muscles during sleep obstructs or partially obstructs the airway. In addition to disrupting sleep for you and your partner at night, it can result in daytime complications such as narcolepsy, the sudden onset of sleep during normal waking hours. Sleep apnea may be linked to obesity, as an accumulation of abdominal fat produces another impediment to adequate breath intake.

If you suspect that you or your partner might have sleep apnea, do not hesitate to check it out. It may be nothing more than a partial nasal blockage, but it could have life-threatening consequences. Attending a sleep clinic will allow experts to observe both your sleep pattern and your brain waves during sleep. Sleep apnea can be the root cause of many problems, from general fatigue to high blood pressure, and high levels of stress hormones that effect blood sugars.

If sleep apnea is diagnosed, continuous positive airway pressure provides some people with simple, helpful relief. You may also wish to explore the possibility of a reduction in the overlapping tissues at the back of the throat with an ear, nose, and throat surgeon.

Whether the issue is simply preparing for a good night's sleep, having a secure and properly conducive environment for sleep, or having sleep apnea, the good news is that all of these circumstances can be improved or fixed.

SEXUAL FITNESS

Diabetes affects both the nerves and the blood supply to the genital organs, impacting the ability to sense and respond to sexual stimuli. Because sexual activity can have an impact on emotional health, normal sexual functioning should be one of our goals in an active, healthy lifestyle. And a good diet and exercise program is your first line of defense in preserving sexual functioning. It can keep arteries open and protect nerves from the degenerating effects of uncontrolled blood sugar.

For men, difficulty maintaining or getting an erection (erectile dysfunction or impotence) is worrisome, both because it is emotionally painful and because it may be an indication of some underlying physical problem. Fortunately, discussion of erectile dysfunction is becoming more public, making it easier for men to take up this issue with their health care providers. Although there are medications such as Viagra on the market for treating erectile dysfunction, be especially careful if you suffer from heart disease, especially if you take heart medication containing nitroglycerin in any form. Using Viagra while taking nitroglycerin can result in a significant loss of blood pressure, and even death, so the risk is certainly not worth the possibility of enhanced sexual functioning.

For women, a lack of libido (sexual urge) can also be a result of diabetes or medications taken for diabetes or depression. Often it may simply take a woman with diabetes longer to climax than before or take more stimulation. Healthy experimentation in one's sex life in the context of a safe and supportive relationship will often go a long way to resolving a lack of libido.

Be sure to examine all the medications you are taking for any condition, as sexual functioning can be compromised by a number of prescription drugs. As a last resort, medications can also be used to enhance sexual activity, but be sure to discuss the risks with a health care provider. Remember that the best way to enhance sexual pleasure is by adopting an active lifestyle, maintaining a healthy weight, eating a nutritious diet, and, of course, having a healthy, supportive, and honest relationship with your partner.

EMOTIONAL FITNESS

No matter how we change the other components of our lifestyle, active living will enhance every part of what we do. We'll be better able to maintain a healthy appetite and resist overeating. It will also help foster a healthy attitude and manage stress, allowing us to remain calm in the face of challenges and burn off stress hormones so that we are more easily able to be kind to those around us.

Stress management is probably the most overlooked component to defeating diabetes, and yet it is one of the most important. Some people use overeating as a way to fight stress, and stress can lead one to feel lethargic and tired. With overweight and inactivity being the tandem contributors to type 2 diabetes, stress must be recognized as an important trigger of these contributors and a focus for any diabetes treatment plan. There are two aspects to stress management: one is protective and the other is proactive.

In the fast-paced world we live in, stress has become a fact of life. We work longer hours, spend less time with our families, eat more hurried meals, travel at faster speeds. Even if things are going well in our lives, our bodies and minds are suffering from increased demands. It would serve us well to develop protective habits as a defense against the everyday stress we encounter and to help us become more calm.

Meyer Friedman, MD, was the first practitioner to identify type A personalities—intense, somewhat aggressive individuals who see the world as a hostile place. Interestingly enough, this phenomenon was actually discovered by Meyer Friedman's upholsterer. This observant gentleman was repairing the chairs in Dr. Friedman's waiting room and discovered an unusual pattern of wear on the upholstery. He stated to Dr. Friedman, a cardiologist, that the people in his waiting room must be the most impatient individuals in the world, as they selectively wore out the fronts and the arms of the chairs in which they sat. Eventually, Dr. Friedman linked this trait of personality, which he termed "type A" or a driven personality, to those at special risk for the development of heart disease. In time, this concept was refined to include the significance of hostility as a particularly damaging aspect of this driven personality type, seeing the world as a hostile place with everyone as a competitor. In several studies, especially of heart disease risk in women, the level of anger and hostility that a person harbors was a strong determinant of their risk for cardiovascular disease. Because heart disease is such a great concern for people with diabetes, monitoring stress can be as important as monitoring blood sugar.

Protecting Your Emotional Health

There are many age-old techniques for calming the mind. Besides hatha yoga, which focuses on strength and flexibility, there are other types of yoga practice that can be revitalizing. For instance, pranayama is a series of breathing techniques that energizes the body and helps bring about a sense of serenity and well-being.

Meditation (and its spiritual adjunct, prayer) teaches how to focus the mind in directions that quiet and soothe the senses. An example of the practical use of meditation can be found in the book *Relaxation Response* by Herbert Benson, a Harvard University PhD. In his studies, auto and factory workers could reduce stress levels and measurably lower their blood pressures simply by focusing their attention for a few minutes a day on a nonsense syllable, in Benson's case, the word "one." Workers in the study group would sit for ten minutes in a quiet place and repeat the word "one" slowly to themselves, imagining that they were dropping a small pebble into a still pond and seeing ripples flowing outward from the pond's surface where the pebble hit. The effects on their blood pressures were dramatic, and with some practice the workers were able to keep their blood pressures and pulse rates lower even after this meditative practice. There's no doubt that such a practice would give significant results to diabetes sufferers with high blood pressure, as well.

In our Steps to Self-Care checklist on pages 162-68, you'll find some tips to help you evaluate how you're handling life's challenges and give you more tools for turning difficult situations into manageable ones. Whichever tool you use, relaxation, like exercise, is something that must be practiced on a daily basis in order to gain the most benefits. The rewards are many, and the calm demeanor that you develop will allow you to become a model of serenity to others.

Creating an Emotionally Healthful Environment

Having a psychological reserve of calmness will allow you to practice kindness. By projecting kindness we can affect the level of stress that surrounds us. If we can transform potentially stressful situations and defuse them, we can take a proactive stance and reduce stress before it touches us.

It's common knowledge that giving makes you feel good; in fact, recent research shows a possible connection between caring for others and a lower incidence of heart disease. Kindness not only does the heart good, it does the body good as well. In terms of objective measures, the levels of stress hormones that rise when we place ourselves in a competitive mindset are marked by elevations of blood sugar. The adrenal gland pours out adrenaline and cortisol over time and predisposes us to insulin resistance. Not only will the dangerous effects of this hormone affect our internal organs, the adrenal glands themselves will be less able to support us when we need a legitimate burst of hormonal support during stress.

One of the most basic concepts of stress management maintains that how we perceive events around us will determine their impact on us. If something is seen as a threat, it affects us deeply; but if we feel we have some control over the situation and can shape our destiny, our level of emotional and physiologic stress is diminished. The determining factor is having a center of control within oneself, a sense of being the captain of one's fate. It requires being able to live life in the moment, dealing with each circumstance as it arises with an optimism that looks for meaning even in the face of adversity. It is an internal perspective and one that we can shape.

The principal skill you need to do a better job of taking life as it comes is the ability to focus attention and attitude, to develop a laserlike mindfulness that can be pulled away from the negative aspects of a situation toward a meaningful and positive view. The development of this skill is not necessarily easy, but it does involve remarkably simple steps.

Imagine a scenario where you're standing in line at the bank, and the person behind you is tapping their foot and looking at their watch, obviously impatient. You could react with annoyance yourself, increasing your stress and hostility level as you observe the other person's impatience. Or you could save your heart some trouble and simply say to the person, "You know, I am not in a hurry, why don't you go ahead?" Where you might have been impatient, you can express love and compassion for another's discomfort and, in the process, have engaged the personal science of healing that comes from an empathic attitude. The newest research on the effect of personality types on heart disease risk in men, for example, stresses that for the typical type A personality (the type of person who is driven to succeed), the greatest likelihood of heart disease will occur in those type As who are not only driven, but also hostile, especially if they are impatient in the process.

One of the nicest ways to achieve a level of calm detachment while dealing with life's challenges was taught by Sri Eknath Easwaran, PhD, a mystic from India who became a professor of English literature at the University of California at Berkeley. An important component of Easwaran's philosophy is that we are not islands unto ourselves; we depend on each other, and how we treat others and the world we live in ultimately affects how we are treated. Easwaran maintained that there is an intimate connection between how well we understand our place in the universe and how much we show compassion for the natural world and make choices day-to-day that reflect this compassion. Easwaran amplified the power of Benson's work on concentrating attention by promoting a focus on inspirational passages rather than meaningless syllables. This not only develops a focused mind, but elevates a sense of personal purpose and self-image.

A particular Buddhist practice is to sit down to every meal with gratitude in our hearts, reflecting this gratitude by looking at each person sitting with us around the table with a smile. We need not be a proverbial "doormat" for the perceived needs of others, but we can practice an attitude of kindness whatever course of action we might choose. Perhaps we cannot allow our teenage son or daughter a certain privilege, but we can do our best to be calm and kind in explaining our decision, offering some alternatives by allowing a certain privilege to be earned.

If we can retrain ourselves to enjoy a lifestyle free of hostility and enmity by focusing our attention on what we can do to help, we can reduce our own risk of illness. Looking at others in a noncompetitive way, with appreciation and a kind eye, frees us to enjoy everyone we meet and see, without hesitation or reservation. "Be kind, be kind, be kind" as a guiding philosophy requires no judgment of others or need for calculation of return. It simply allows for the pleasure of goodwill, which is completely and unreservedly self-enriching.

While we may not be able to return to a life that emulates the extended, enduring family and friendship ties that characterized the past, we can begin to value the kindness and consideration inherent in those values again. And where we are able, we need to imitate them. Without that kindness, the heart disease, immune imbalance, hostility, and anger that run rampant in our culture will be especially injurious to our health.

GUIDE TO LIVING WELL

- Aim for sixty minutes of physical activity each day. Include flexibility, strength, and aerobic exercise in your workout.

- Get adequate sleep. The hours between 10 P.M. and midnight may be the most important of all.

- Recognize changes in your libido. Notice how you feel both physically and emotionally.

- Don't smoke, use excessive amounts of alcohol, or abuse other drugs.

- Work to maintain healthy relationships with your spouse, children, partners, workplace acquaintances, and friends.

- Strive to be happy and radiate happiness to those around you. You will benefit from this attitudinal healing.

- Don't ignore problems, but be proactive with your future, and attempt to fix things before they get broken. Prevention is both less expensive and less difficult to experience than repair.

CHAPTER 9

Self Care: A Daily Maintenance Routine

Now that you have a treatment plan in place and are regularly monitoring your blood sugar, it's time to begin another important part of your care—daily maintenance. All of us should be in the business of caring for ourselves. This is true whether we have a health challenge like insulin resistance or diabetes, or whether we simply are interested in a sensible lifestyle for the maintenance of high-level wellness. But, without a doubt, those of us with diabetes are at increased risk of nearly every major complication that we would normally face, so a helpful self-care checklist used daily can be a real life saver. For example, a person with diabetes and without known heart disease has a risk of heart attack and sudden cardiac death equal to a nondiabetic person of the same age who has had a heart attack. As well, diabetes raises one's risk of eye disease, kidney disease, nerve damage, autoimmune disease, dental problems, infections, and arterial disease resulting in a stroke. Therefore, not only are the lifestyle changes we have emphasized in this book vital, they are especially important if you have diabetes and need to recognize problems before they become something to worry about.

An honest daily self-care routine employs a dose of common sense, combined with a genuine interest in one's own being. Our bodies and minds are marvelous tools and wonderful machines which require, in general, fairly minimal maintenance. But a little attention now and again is warranted and pays off big dividends. Did you ever want to win the lottery? Well, all of the lottery money in the world will not purchase a return of your health, once you have lost it. Our health is our most precious possession. And we can protect it with simple daily routines and choices.

Before going on to the details of the daily safety check, let us take a moment to remind ourselves of two very powerful facts. First, smoking is a disaster for the health of any human being, and most especially for those with diabetes, and second, excessive use of alcohol is harmful. The mortality risk associated with smoking is simply a rising straight line until a certain threshold of exposure is reached, then the risk rises exponentially. Even secondhand exposure is deadly, as evidenced by the mortality and poor health suffered by the spouses and children of smokers.

Alcohol intake is more complicated. While the excessive use of alcohol is the leading preventable cause of fatal motor vehicle accidents, and while if wrongly used, alcohol intake ruins lives and relationships, it must be said that with control and moderation, alcohol can improve cardiovascular health. One drink a day for women, and one or two a day for men, has been associated in the largest epidemiological studies that we have analyzed with a decrease in mortality from heart attack and stoke. Clearly, this assessment of risk versus benefit varies from person to person; however, it is very clear that excessive alcohol intake is harmful.

Your Daily Safety Checklist—Steps to Self-Care

Start the day and end the day with a safety check. In the still quiet of the morning, perhaps getting up with a few minutes to spare so you are not rushed, run a quick inventory check of "all systems." Begin by taking several deep breaths, training yourself to expand the abdomen, then bring the breath up into the chest and expand it fully. Finally, lift the collar bones a fraction of an inch for the fullest inhalation. Hold your breath at the point of greatest expansion of the chest cavity, then slowly release it through pursed lips, closing the back of the throat a little so that there is a bit of a hissing sound. It will sound as if you were breathing through a "Darth Vadar" mask, with a slight resistance to the exhalation and a slight hiss in the back of the throat. In general, breathe in through the nose to warm and condition the air entering the lungs, so that the ciliated nasal cells can remove bacteria and other contaminants in the process.

Breath control is closely associated with evenness of temper and emotion as well, so practicing full, even breaths is cleansing both in terms of physiology and emotion. It is a beneficial way to both start and end the day. Often, especially as people become less aware of their physical condition, they forget how important it is to breathe fully and deeply, and eventually may lose that capacity. So, remind your body and mind how important your vital capacity really is and prevent the development of restrictive lung disease by this simple self-maintenance tool. Now, you are ready to begin.

☑ MUSCLES AND JOINTS

Any areas where muscles are tight? Any pain in the joints, any swelling? Think back over the last few days; are any joints particularly bothersome? Pain in the knees when going up stairs, etc.? If so, look at ways of reducing stress on that joint. For example, if you are overweight and have problems with your hips, knees, feet, or ankles, then losing weight may be a major part of the solution. Certainly, having high insulin levels does raise the risk of joint inflammation where there may be some wear and tear, and a change in diet toward plant-based foods will lessen this inflammation, even while it helps you with weight management. The most common form of degenerative joint disease is osteoarthritis, a degrading of the protective cartilage that cushions the impact of bone on bone in the joints. This cartilage allows stability with flexibility, working with the structure of the ligaments and tendons that hold the joint structures together. As we age, we may notice some broadening of the finger joints, along with stiffness, especially in the morning. Maybe our safety check will reveal a particular pattern of wear on a joint so that we can review what activity we are doing that may contribute to the problem. In general, exercise is actually beneficial for joints afflicted by osteoarthritis. However if we are putting specific repetitive strain on a particular joint, we should consider changing the pattern of activity that we recognize as damaging, wherever possible.

On the other hand, if you notice red, hot, swollen joints, especially if this process is persistent and symmetrical, that is, involving the same joints on both sides of the body (both knees or both wrists), you may be suffering from an autoimmune or infectious arthritis, such as rheumatic arthritis. Depending on exposure and location, the possibility of arthritis related to Lyme disease from a tick bite should also be considered. In either case, your personal physician should be consulted to give you an informed diagnosis.

The nonweight-bearing joints, such as the elbows and shoulders, should be checked for range of motion, noticing any restriction or pain, and the skin and the shape of the joint should also look normal. Anything out of the ordinary should be addressed with exercise or massage. If the situation worsens, check with your physician; it is important to prevent the joint from stiffening, as that will require more dramatic intervention.

☑ EYES AND EARS

Is your vision crisp and clear, and equal on both sides? Unfortunately, diabetic retinopathy (damage to the retina of the eye) is one of the more serious complications of high blood sugar and high blood pressure over a long period of time, as it damages the tiny blood vessels of the eyes. We know that the better blood sugar is controlled, the less the damage there will be to the retina. If damage does occur, it is best discovered and treated early, so it's important to see an eye specialist who can check your eyes every six months. In many cases, there are laser therapies that will stop the damage before it gets too severe. However, the best treatment continues to be prevention—keeping blood sugars as close to normal as possible.

Other very common eye problems seen in people with diabetes are cataracts and glaucoma. Cataracts may initially impair night vision, making driving more dangerous. They appear like a haze in the lens of the eye and can be caused by high blood sugars or oxidative damage from sunlight. Smoking and poor diet both accelerate cataract development. Cataracts are easily repairable and should be treated promptly. Protect yourself by practicing good diabetic control, eating a diet rich in antioxidants, and wearing protective sunglasses to prevent overexposure to strong ultraviolet (UV) rays.

Glaucoma is the result of pressure building in the eye that damages the optic nerve. Initially, it causes loss of peripheral vision, so you have trouble seeing to the side when you are looking straight ahead. Glaucoma is a progressive disease and requires correction, or it puts you at risk of early blindness!

Another common vision problem is macular degeneration, the most common cause of blindness in the developed world. It used to be considered an inevitable disease of aging. Now we know it is related to a lack of protective phytochemicals in the diet over a lifetime. As we mentioned in chapter 3, colorful fruits and vegetables contain secondary nutrients, like zeaxanthin and lutein. These yellow and orange pigments concentrate in the macula, the central focusing area of the retina. There is scientific evidence to suggest that an antioxidant-rich diet can even curb macular degeneration after it has begun, especially if the disease is recognized early. You may want to supplement with a multivitamin that contains lutein in order to get additional ocular protection. Prevention of light-related damage to this area of the eye is also critical, as this is where vision is most acute and sharp.

Have an eye professional who is experienced with diabetes examine your eyes at least yearly, more often if necessary. Eye diseases from diabetes are the leading cause of blindness in North America, so they must be taken very seriously. Watch for blurry or double vision, dark or floating spots, or flashing light that appears to some people like lightning. Flashes may be a sign of detachment of the retinal membrane, a serious condition that needs immediate medical care. If you feel pain or pressure in your eyes or begin to notice your peripheral vision disappearing, visit your eye doctor!

Is your hearing good? The eighth cranial nerve, which is responsible for hearing, is also involved with balance. It can be affected by aging and diabetic nerve damage, so any change there should be addressed early. Ringing in the ears, or tinnitus, is both bothersome and a potentially worrisome sign Why is it so worrisome? if associated with hearing loss in one ear, since it may indicate a rare but dangerous cancerous tumor of the acoustic nerve. Usually tinnitus is the result of high-frequency hearing loss from noise exposure over the years, but requires careful checking to rule out more serious problems. There are good options available to treat even severe hearing loss, so check any hearing difficulties you might have with your physician or audiologist. Don't just grin and bear it!

☑ Skin and Hair

Take the time to note the condition of your scalp, hair, and skin. Is the skin dry and flaky, or full of moisture and resilience? If you notice changes, first check to see that the soaps, shampoos, and cosmetics you're using are gentle and free of detergents (like sodium lauryl sulfate) and coloring agents and preservatives, such as diethanolamine (DEA), which has been linked to cancer. Ideally, use only the simplest, natural products with the fewest ingredients, as contaminants in these preparations are absorbed through the skin and are potentially harmful. If the scalp is red or bleeding, or there is hair loss, especially in defined round areas, check with your physician. Persistent sores may represent skin cancer, and areas of hair loss may be a sign of a scalp fungal infection or an autoimmune disease called alopecia areata. Both of these may be more common in people with diabetes, so they should be checked by your physician.

Is the skin too oily, bordering on greasy? The incidence of thyroid disease is higher with diabetes, and this might promote excess oil on the skin and hair. Is your complexion rosy or pale? If flushed, consider infection or hormonal changes with midlife, or a reaction to some food. If pale, consider anemia or a lack of iron, and be sure there is a good reason for your anemic condition. Unexplained anemia, in the absence of menstruation or accidental blood loss or surgery, must be considered a sign of underlying serious disease. Have your red blood cell count checked; if it is low, find out why.

It's important to protect the skin by keeping it moist and prevent cracking that may lead to infection. When blood sugar is high, the skin tends to be drier, putting you at risk for sores that are difficult to heal. Keep your skin moist and supple, especially on exposed areas such as hands and particularly the feet. (See more in the foot care section that follows.) Use simple almond, grape seed, or olive oil as a healthful stimulating massage and to seal water into the outer layer of skin, to help it maintain integrity. These oils are available in pharmacies, groceries, and health food stores, and are valuable and benign to the skin. Do not heavily coat the skin, but lightly burnish the skin with a brisk rub, invigorating the circulation, superficially and finally, deeply, especially where there are areas that are tight or tender. If you wish, add a tiny amount, a few drops, of an essential oil, such as lavender, rosemary, or rosewood. Do not overuse the essential oil either, and be sure to choose something you associate with good memories and that brings you strength.

☑ Feet

Now, focus on your feet. When you have diabetes, your elevated blood sugar literally bathes the nerves and vital organs of the body in a sweetened, syrupy blood and lymph fluid. This results in injury to the nerves, especially the longest nerves of the body, in the legs. As a result, you may not feel damage or injury to your feet that may have occurred during the day. As well, tiny arteries carrying immune cells to the periphery of the body become clogged with arterial plaque, so the possibility of infection is increased. Also, watch for the development of athlete's foot, a common condition that occurs when feet sweat in shoes or boots, creating a perfect atmosphere for the growth of fungal infections.

At the beginning and end of every day, massage the soles of your feet with your thumbs, separating the toes and moving them through a full range of motion. Take special note of any wounds, cracked skin, or redness (and upward spread of that redness) which might mark an early infection. After a bath or shower, liberally apply body oil to damp skin to seal in moisture. Petroleum products and silicones may be absorbed through the skin, so choose natural plant oils that have been cold pressed and are free of solvents and preservatives. If you are at all concerned by any problem, have it looked at by a physician, podiatrist, or your health care provider as soon as possible.

☑ Mouth, Teeth, and Gums

Look at your mouth, teeth, and gums. Floss and brush your teeth carefully at least daily, ideally twice a day. Are your gums red, sore, or swollen? Do they bleed when you brush them? Are your gums pulling away from your teeth? While dental diseases are very common for everyone, people with diabetes experience more of these problems, especially if blood sugar control is poor. High blood sugar encourages the growth of bacteria, increasing plaque buildup on your teeth. This contributes to redness, swelling, and bleeding of gums.

As well, there can be a greater incidence of dry mouth resulting from a lack of saliva. Since saliva protects against bacterial growth, this can be a cause for concern. If you notice an increase in dry mouth, be sure that you are not dehydrated, as many of us, especially those of us with high blood sugar, do not drink enough water. Water intake is remarkably protective, so it is vital to include a review of water intake in your safety check. Ideally, drink six to ten glasses of pure, clean water daily. Finally, dry mouth may be an indication not only of poor blood sugar control, but also of an underlying autoimmunity disorder affecting the salivary glands. If this is a persisting issue for you, see your health care provider.

If you wear false teeth, it is important to keep them clean too. And remember that with false teeth, you don't often feel objects like bones or poorly chewed chunks of food that may cause either pain or obstruction when swallowed. So, take the time to thoroughly chew your food, whether or not you have your own "chompers." The process of digestion, and indeed the quality of your saliva itself, is influenced by how well you chew your food.

☑ *Stress Level*

ike our IQ, or intelligence quotient, we have an SQ, a stress quotient, that measures our ability to handle stress. What tools are there for assessment of our stress quotient?

1) Your personal stress monitor. Do a self-check for stress every day, especially in the early morning just on arising and just before retiring in the evening. When you first wake up, what comes to your mind? Are you angry, upset, or worried about something? Write it down and address it that day if possible. Consider the worst-case scenario. Then allow yourself to devise a game plan for that worst case, understanding that, in all likelihood, nothing that bad will happen. Then remember to always end your self-stress monitoring session with a list of three things for which you are thankful and grateful!

Just before retiring, think of the day with gratitude, and also write down any unfinished business, promising yourself that you will take care of these issues the very next day. Not all unfinished business will be resolved the next day, but you can begin to address the issues. Often, during the night, your unconscious mind's vast resources will come up with a solution.

2) Your relationship focus. Again, for a moment on awakening and just before retiring, think about your closest relationships. Are there any things left unsaid or undone? If so, when can they be said or done? The sooner the better! It is enriching, enlightening, and healing to address issues as soon as they are in your mind's eye. And remember, be positive, be positive, be positive. There is an ancient wisdom that states that before anything is actually said, a statement would have to pass three gates: is it true; is it kind; is it necessary? Once those criteria are fulfilled, then perhaps the comment is worth sharing with others. That having been said, the key to reducing stress in a relationship is to communicate, constantly, relentlessly, and honestly.

3) Lowering the stress level. Applying the practical tools of meditation and relaxation for a few minutes a day will provide a resiliency of body and that will serve you well. Repeat a favorite prayer slowly in your mind, allowing each word to drop from your thought into the calm space in your mind's eye, as if it were a pearl dropping into a still pond. Allow enough time between the words of the passage for a few "ripples" to flow outward from the first word before adding the second. Slowly work your way through the passage. If your mind strays, bring it back. The practical results of this type of practice are a remarkable reserve of strength and the ability to handle the challenges of life with aplomb.

CHAPTER 10

When Diet & Exercise Are Not Enough

T here are some cases where diabetes cannot be adequately controlled with diet and exercise. Perhaps at the time of initial diagnosis of diabetes, blood sugar levels are extremely high. The priority in that situation would be to bring these levels down quickly using whichever treatments are effective. Also, your diabetes may have already progressed to a level where you'll need the support of insulin or other medications in order to keep blood sugar under control. At that point a number of other treatment options, in addition to diet and exercise, need to be explored. The next step might be to add oral medications to either increase the output of insulin or restore the body's inherent sensitivity to its own insulin. If diet, exercise, and oral medications fail to be effective, insulin by injection is generally advised.

169

It is important to note that the use of medications is neither necessarily safe nor is it the best approach for young people who are increasingly at risk and suffering from insulin resistance in even greater numbers. As is true with any medication, there can be adverse effects from years and years of exposure. Even though oral medications may seem to be the easy alternative to making diet and lifestyle changes, there can be a steep price to pay in the long run.

When conventional therapies do not provide the desired results or have unacceptable side effects, alternative therapies are often considered. Even though they are not often practiced in hospitals or diabetes clinics, they offer a viable option. Among the most popular alternative therapies used in the management of diabetes have been acupuncture, biofeedback, guided imagery, vitamin and mineral supplementation, and the use of herbal and botanical preparations. While many of these therapies have shown promise, most are either untested or unproven based on current scientific standards. They do, however, have a long cultural tradition in societies around the world, and when one looks at their benefits, at least in terms of individuals or pilot studies, they show promise. Even though it might be difficult to design a study for assessing alternative techniques that would pass muster with modern Western scientific standards, these methods are worth exploring.

The biggest concern about recommending alternative therapies is that you might choose to give up conventional therapies that are working to control your blood sugar in favor of something more "natural" or "herbal." Never forget that natural herbs are drugs, just like drugs from the drug store, only you don't need a prescription for them. There are other concerns about botanicals, herbs, and other alternative therapies, such as the lack of control in their preparations, the lack of widely accepted certification for many of the alternative practitioners, and our lack of knowledge about how these treatments will combine with conventional medications. For example, there was a recent case of an elderly man on insulin who added ginseng to his treatment regimen and suffered a serious hypoglycemic episode. Studies done at the University of Toronto do show that ginseng has a potent hypoglycemic effect. So all caution must be advised in combining a botanical like ginseng with traditional medications for glucose control.

Whatever you choose to investigate, be sure to inform your health care team about any changes or choices you are thinking of making when it comes to controlling your diabetes.

THE ORAL MEDICATIONS

O ral medications might be needed to stimulate beta cells in the pancreas to pour out more insulin, especially at times when blood glucose levels are high, such as after a meal. They might also be needed to increase insulin sensitivity, usually in combination with efforts to reduce the amount of carbohydrate in one's diet. These medications, often called "oral hypoglycemic agents," can be divided into five broad categories.

- Sulfonylureas
- Biguanides
- Alpha-glucosidase inhibitors
- Thiozolidinediones
- Meglitinides

As in the case of all medications, each category has its advantages and disadvantages. Different drugs can be combined to realize the strengths of each and achieve optimal control. However, any time a new type of treatment is added to your diabetes control regimen, the risk for low blood sugar, or hypoglycemia, may increase.

The Sulfonylureas The sulfonylureas are a mainstay in the management of blood sugar in people with diabetes. This category of medications, sold under a variety of brand names, work by stimulating the pancreas to make more insulin and helping the body better use the insulin it makes. However, the sulfonylureas can cause weight gain and many individuals who are allergic to the sulfa class of antibiotics (such as the often prescribed Septra or Bactrim) may also be reactive to the sulfonylureas. Also, these medications often cause swings of blood sugar and symptoms of low blood sugar (hypoglycemia) to occur, especially in the elderly. Newer sulfonylureas are less likely than older types such as chlorpropamide to cause long-lasting low blood sugar in the elderly, a condition which can lead to despondency and depression. Still, you need to be vigilant about the very real risks that episodes of hypoglycemia, or low blood sugar, can pose, as it can be life-threatening in both the short and the long term.

The Biguanides The biguanide medications were initially thought to provide a means of restoring lost insulin sensitivity. However, it's more likely that they reduce the amount of glucose released by the liver from the storage starches kept there (called glycogen). The advantage of biguanides is that they only rarely cause low blood sugar reactions. As well, they are often useful in promoting weight loss, especially in older people. Anyone using insulin but who still has difficulty controlling their blood sugar will often benefit from the addition of one of the biguanides.

However, the biguanides are also occasionally hazardous, especially in people with poor kidney function. They can cause a dangerous increase in the accumulation of lactic acid in the body, which worsens kidney function, contributes to metabolic acidosis, and ultimately leads to death. With wise use these problems are rare, but vigilance is required. For people with impaired kidney function, other drugs, such as ACE inhibitors and angiotensin receptor blockers (ARBs), should be considered.

The Thiozolidinediones   The newest medications for glucose control, the thiozolidinediones, have become very popular for restoring insulin sensitivity. The newer members of this category are well tolerated and relatively safe, although quite expensive. The medications are often used in the earliest stages of insulin resistance to rebalance the body's ability to utilize insulin. There are early indications that the thiozolidinediones might cause excessive sodium retention and heart failure in those suffering from severe diabetes.

The Alpha-Glucosidase Inhibitors   Alpha-glucosidase inhibitors block enzymes that digest starches. This action causes a slower, lower rise in blood sugar, especially after meals, without causing blood sugar to drop too low. One of the problems with drugs that block carbohydrate breakdown and absorption in the intestine is that bloating and gas in the colon can occur. This discomfort usually diminishes with time. The alpha-glucosidase inhibitors do not usually cause other side effects, such as low blood sugar.

The Meglitinides   The meglitinides are a relatively new family of diabetes medications. This family stimulates the pancreas to make more insulin. In doing so, it helps reduce blood sugar after eating. They seem to be well tolerated, although our experience with them is limited. Meglitinides are best used as single agents early in the course of diabetes, when fasting blood sugars may still be normal but rises in glucose and triglycerides after meals are a problem. There do not appear to be any side effects, such as gastrointestinal distress or low blood sugar reactions.

INJECTABLE INSULIN

Sometimes in type 2 diabetes, high levels of insulin are circulating in the body but sensitivity to that insulin is decreasing. In this case, injectable insulin will be prescribed. Insulin might also be used along with other drugs to restore sensitivity to insulin, as in the "bedtime insulin, daytime oral meds" approach.

These synthetic, injectable insulins are identical to the natural insulin that our bodies produce, so they don't tend to cause allergic responses. However, in a sad way, adding insulin when the body's own insulin levels are already high is, in effect, adding fuel to a metabolic fire of increasing inflammation, and increasing the risk for hardening of the arteries, as well as obesity. Insulin is a growth hormone and meant to promote storage of calories, so when insulin levels are high, the body becomes more efficient at absorbing nutrients from the food we eat into our fat and glycogen stores. When insulin levels are chronically high, the tendency to gain weight is significant. One has to balance the use of insulin for glycemic control with the possibility of weight gain, which in and of itself tends to increase insulin resistance and worsen blood sugar control.

According to Dr. Anne Kenshole, a prominent diabetologist at the University of Toronto, when insulin is added to a diabetes management program, it also causes weight gain simply by stopping the loss of glucose in the urine. In other words, the added insulin enhances glucose utilization, reducing the elimination of glucose that sometimes causes weight loss and wasting seen in people before they are properly diagnosed with diabetes. For example, patients in one study given insulin over a ten-year period gained more weight than subjects on therapy with oral medications. There is also a concern with rising insulin levels, whether natural or injected, being associated with increased deaths from cardiovascular disease. In people who do not have diabetes, rising insulin levels do correlate with increased heart attack rates. Studies are underway that will provide better answers to concerns about rising insulin and potential heart problems.

TIMING YOUR MEALS WITH YOUR MEDICATIONS

The timing of meals is an important consideration for people on insulin and/or sulfonylurea medications. If you delay a meal when you are on these medications, your blood sugar could dip too low and you could become hypoglycemic.

If your meal is delayed by about an hour, there is generally little cause for concern, unless you are using a rapid-acting insulin. If you usually take your medication or insulin before the meal you delay, you will simply be taking it a little later. You may wish to delay your other meals by about a half hour each as well. Otherwise, you may need to have a small snack at your usual mealtime (for example, a starch or a fruit). Also, if you are using a very long-acting insulin as a baseline medication given at night (such as Ultralente or the newer glargine long-acting insulin) these generally will not have to be adjusted unless there is a very long delay in eating.

If your meal is delayed one and a half hours or more, you will need to consider your options. The best choice for you depends on how often you take insulin and/or sulfonylurea diabetes pills.

Timing of Insulin or Sulfonylureas

Morning only:

The simplest course of action is to eat the snack that would normally follow the delayed meal at the usual time of the meal. For example, if you delay your usual 12:00 lunch to 2:00 P.M., eat your afternoon snack at 12:00.

Before breakfast and before dinner (using a mixture of short-acting insulin and intermediate-acting insulin [NPH or lente], premixed insulin [70/30], or sulfonylureas):

You have two options if on sulfonylureas (options 1 or 2), and three if on insulin (options 1-3):

1. Take your insulin or pills as usual before your normal evening meal time, but eat your evening snack at your usual mealtime. For example, if your usual dinner time is at 6:00, but tonight's dinner is delayed until 7:30, you would take your insulin or sulfonylurea at your usual time (around 5:30), and eat your evening snack at 6:00.

2. Wait until thirty minutes before the delayed meal to take your insulin or medication. Have your evening snack before bed (or if the meal is a drawn-out affair, add your snack allowance to your dinner and omit the evening snack). For example, if your dinner is delayed until 8:00 and your usual mealtime is 6:00, take your insulin at 7:30.

3. Split the dose around the delayed meal into two shots. For example, if dinner is delayed, you could take your intermediate-acting insulin at your usual dinnertime (it won't start acting for one to two hours) and your short-acting insulin thirty minutes before you eat. At your regular mealtime, you should eat a snack providing about 15 grams of carbohydrate (e.g., a starch or fruit).

Before meals (use of rapid-acting (humalog/lispro/aspart) or short-acting (regular) insulin before all meals):

If you take rapid-acting insulin (Humalog/lispro/aspart), do so just before you eat. If on short-acting (regular) insulin, take it 30 minutes before you eat the delayed meal. If your blood sugar dips too low before the delayed meal, eat about 15 grams of carbohydrate (e.g., a starch or fruit).

No matter how careful you are about compensating for meal delays, things can go awry, so be prepared! Your dinner companions could be delayed in traffic, your reservation lost, or your chef very slow. Thus, it is important to always carry some convenient carbohydrate source with you. Dried fruits, fresh fruits, granola bars, crackers, juice, or candy will all do the trick. Keep such snacks handy in your car, desk, purse, or briefcase in case of an emergency. Also, don't be afraid to explain to the management or the server at the restaurant just why it is that you are concerned about the timing of your meal.

ALTERNATIVE APPROACHES

While not a cure or treatment for diabetes, acupuncture, biofeedback, and guided imagery may be useful in reducing both the stress associated with normal metabolic functions (such as oxidation) and hormonal stress, both of which directly oppose the action of insulin in our bodies. Reducing these stresses will help achieve better glucose control. These methods can also have an important role in treating the pain associated with nerve damage caused by diabetes.

Acupuncture is an ancient science with its roots in China. It is founded on the principle that with good health there is a free flow of energy (Qi, pronounced chee) throughout the body and between the body's organs. Ancient Chinese science theorized the existence of a network of energy channels in the body, called meridians, through which Qi flows. The theory is that when Qi is free to move about the body, then good health and well-being are maintained. Acupuncture involves a procedure in which a practitioner inserts a very slender sterilized needle into special points of the skin to stimulate the meridians and release the flow of energy, relieving pain and promoting healing. As an alternative to needles, sometimes heat or cold, pressure, small gold or silver pellets, electrical stimulation, or a low-intensity laser device is used to achieve the same results.

Biofeedback is a simple technique that teaches stress management through relaxation, helping people better deal with the pain associated with nerve damage. With biofeedback you are trained to control the blood flow to one hand, the level of muscular tension throughout the body, or to reduce your heart rate to achieve a deep state of relaxation. This has the effect of reducing stress hormone levels, blood pressure, pain levels, and even the severity of impairment in heart disease and severe lung disease.

Guided imagery is also a useful relaxation technique that teaches people to focus on positive, healing images. Often guided imagery is designed not only to engender a relaxation response, but also to promote a targeted immune response. For example, one might imagine valiant immune cells of the body searching out and destroying any tumor cells that might be present. In the work of pioneers like Dr. Bernie Seigel or Dr. Carl Simonton, these techniques were used in combination with other treatment methods to help maintain metabolism, limit tumor growth, and achieve a better sense of well-being or quality of life. Although guided imagery has been used as a healing technique by many cultures through history, only a small number of scientific studies have shown its effectiveness.

NUTRITIONAL SUPPLEMENTS

While the thought of nutritional supplements impacting blood sugar control may seem surprising, there is some evidence suggesting that their use could be beneficial. The supplements that have received the most attention are chromium, magnesium, vanadium taurine, and alpha-lipoic acid.

Chromium is the supplement most often recognized as beneficial for people with diabetes, although its use has been hotly debated in the scientific community. Several studies have suggested that chromium improves control of diabetes, because it is needed to make "glucose tolerance factor," a substance which helps improve insulin function. There have been two important Chinese studies showing that chromium supplementation has beneficial effects on glycemic control. Other, larger studies have not gotten similar results. Currently, no formal recommendations for chromium supplementation exist for people with diabetes. However, researchers who have studied chromium in the human diet feel most people are deficient in this mineral and would likely benefit from some supplementation in modest amounts. Chromium is present in nuts, seeds, and whole grains. The addition of a modest amount of chromium in a supplement would likely be beneficial in helping to control blood sugar.

Magnesium deficiency has been linked by several studies to an increased risk of type 2 diabetes. Magnesium helps relax muscles and conduct nerve impulses, and activates many of the body's enzymes to complete chemical reactions. Studies have shown that a lack of magnesium reduces the secretion of insulin by the pancreas and increases insulin resistance in body tissues. In addition, people with type 2 diabetes who were given magnesium supplements improved short-term insulin response and glycemic control. More than 80 percent of the magnesium is lost from whole grains when they are milled, and it is not added back when flour is enriched. Legumes, nuts, seeds, whole grains, dark, leafy green vegetables, and bananas are good sources of magnesium.

Vanadium is a trace mineral found in miniscule amounts in plants and animals. A recent study found that vanadium supplementation produced modest increases in insulin sensitivity and a slight reduction in insulin requirements. However, the evidence is slight, and the best that can be said is that we could all benefit by eating a variety of whole foods on a regular basis. These foods would provide not just vanadium, but many other important trace elements, such as boron, manganese, and zinc, that are required for numerous enzyme systems throughout the body. Rich sources of vanadium include dill, radishes, eggs, vegetable oils, buckwheat, oats, and peppers.

Taurine is an amino acid that acts as a buffer and protects the cell membranes from damage. Recent research suggests that taurine is also a hypoglycemic agent, enhancing the effects of insulin. Early trials are encouraging, but larger trials are needed before taurine can be recommended as a supplement for people with diabetes.

Alpha-lipoic acid is a sulfur-containing compound, long recognized for its vital role in energy production within the cell, and more recently for its tremendous potential as an antioxidant. It neutralizes free radicals in both the fatty and watery regions of cells, in contrast to vitamin C (which is water soluble) and vitamin E (which is fat soluble). For this reason, it has been nicknamed the "universal" antioxidant. Insufficient alpha-lipoic acid can seriously compromise the effectiveness of other antioxidants, including vitamins C and E. It directly recycles and extends the lifespans of vitamin C and glutathione, and it indirectly renews vitamin E. This unique antioxidant is not considered a vitamin because the body can manufacture adequate amounts; however, there is some evidence that adding to our natural production may have its advantages. Interest in alpha-lipoic acid is increasing rapidly among diabetes researchers. Evidence suggests that it enhances glucose uptake in people with type 2 diabetes, decreases insulin resistance, and repairs nerve damage. Some preliminary data also suggests that it may also improve visual function in people with glaucoma. Alpha-lipoic acid is only found in very small amounts in foods, thus nutritional supplements are generally advised for people wishing to increase intake. Amounts commonly recommended range from approximately 100 to 800 mg per day.

HERBALS AND BOTANICALS

What about herbals and botanicals, those supplements that contain extracts or active ingredients from the roots, berries, seeds, stems, leaves, buds, or flowers of plants? Certainly, there has been intriguing research suggesting herbs such as ginseng and gingko can be helpful in reducing blood sugar levels. The wisdom of both the ancient Indian and Chinese medical systems would suggest that this might be the case. Western medical science has shown that these "tonic herbs" may enhance glucose utilization and are "adaptogenic," providing protection from common age- and stress-related damage that occurs as a natural part of metabolic function, such as oxidation.

If you are considering combining Western medications with botanicals, it is best to proceed cautiously and realize that our understanding of the interactions between drugs and plant substances, while growing, is not clear. Not only are medicines for blood sugar control affected, but blood thinners as well, so caution is definitely advised. Keeping your health practitioners in the loop about any treatment you decide to follow on your own would be essential for your own protection. In order to avoid any possible drug interactions, these botanical approaches are best tried as a supplement to diet and exercise interventions only, and not interventions involving oral diabetes medications or injectable insulin.

MONITORING YOUR BLOOD GLUCOSE LEVELS

The goal of any diabetes treatment method is normal glucose and insulin levels, and normal to near-normal levels of blood fats. Although your health practitioner will want to monitor your progress from time to time, regular self-testing will give you the best sense of how you're doing. Check the glycemic control guidelines in table 10.1 for an interpretation of what various glucose levels mean in terms of what action you'll need to take. Anything less than the "ideal" column (or the column for those already diagnosed with diabetes) leaves you open for a higher risk of complications.

Tools to Monitor Progress

In the past, we relied on urine monitoring to determine if glucose levels were normal. If sugar spilled out through the kidneys, we would measure it with a "dipstick" test done with a glucostix strip. If our body was burning fat and

TABLE 10.1		Guidelines for Glycemic Control in People with Type 2 Diabetes*		

Index	Ideal (nondiabetic)	Goal for those with diabetes	Suboptimal (action suggested)	Inadequate (action required)
Blood Glucose (before meals/ fasting)	68-110 mg/dL	70-120 mg/dL	130-180 mg/dL	over 180 mg/dL
	3.8-6.1 mmol/L	3.9-6.7 mmol/L	7.1-10.0 mmol/L	over 10 mmol/L
Blood Glucose (2 hrs after eating)	80-125 mg/dL	90-180 mg/dL	200-250 mg/dL	over 250 mg/dL
	4.4-7.0 mmol/L	5.0-10 mmol/L	11.1-14 mmol/L	over 14 mmol/L
HbA1c	less than 6	less than 7	more than 7	more than 8

*Adapted from the American Diabetes Association. Position statement: standards of medical care for patients with diabetes mellitus. *Diabetes Care.* 1998:21 (suppl):S24, and Meltzer, S. et al. Clinical Practice Guidelines for the Management of Diabetes in Canada. *Can Med Assoc. J.* 1998; 159 (suppl 8): 159S1.

protein and creating ketones (acidic compounds excreted in the urine), these could be seen on a ketostix urine dip test. Ideally, there should be no sugar in the urine when we are doing well with blood sugar control.

Because some people spill glucose into the urine more easily than others, urine monitoring is not a sensitive or accurate measurement of glucose control for diabetes. Also, now that the technology for measuring glucose levels in a drop of blood has advanced, we can fairly accurately tell what our blood sugar is at the moment with a simple, inexpensive, home-monitoring device called a fingerstick test.

The newest devices are able to estimate blood glucose levels accurately through the skin, without drawing blood, although these are not yet widely available and must be used with regular fingerstick and strip testing.

When to Monitor

If blood sugars are controlled and remain in consistently normal ranges, then home glucose testing once or twice a week should be fine. An additional test can be administered if you are ill, feeling poorly, or the symptoms of excessive thirst, excessive urination, and dry mouth have returned. On the other hand, if blood sugar control is poor, it would be good to monitor daily, or even more frequently, until control is achieved.

With the newer, fast-acting insulins, many people will want to test for blood sugar levels before each meal and at bedtime to adjust their insulin dose. If there's an increase in physical activity, it would be a good idea to test for any signs of low blood sugar to recognize and ward off hypoglycemic symptoms before they might occur.

There is one other valuable test to monitor blood sugar control, the A1c test, which is performed by your health care provider. The A1c test is a way of estimating what your blood sugar control has been over the past three months or so by measuring how much glucose has attached to protein in your red blood cells. The A1c is especially helpful in sorting out difficult control issues, as it gives a big picture look at long-term control over months, rather than an hour-to-hour report that fingerstick tests provide. You should be looking for normal levels of 6 percent or less as an A1c test marker.

If any of your tests indicate problems, you should address these quickly with a health care provider experienced in the medical management of diabetes. Most family physicians and internists can help with routine diabetes management. With special concerns, a specialist in diabetes or endocrinology can be a valuable resource. How often you see your physician or health care provider will depend on how well you are doing, but regular monitoring schedules are important. Plan to see your health care provider a few times a year if you are not perfectly controlled, and more often if control is difficult. A registered dietitian or certified diabetes educator can be helpful and should be sought out for monitoring and clinical support on a regular basis.

In addition to regular blood sugar monitoring, you will want to monitor other indications of diabetes complications, such as eye damage, foot problems, cardiac disease, nerve damage, high blood pressure, and stroke risk. These and any other health concerns should be discussed with your health care team.

A Final Note

One of the biggest issues with blood sugar control is simply denial that there is a problem. Even after a diagnosis of diabetes, there can be a tendency to ignore medical advice, despite the risk of serious trouble. Don't be in denial. Simply being proactive with your own health care greatly reduces your risk for future problems.

CHAPTER 11

Kitchen Wizardry: Tricks of the Trade

Y ou have learned about hydrogenated fats, pro-oxidants, antioxidants and phytochemicals. You have a pretty good idea of the kinds of dietary changes that are required to turn this disease around, and you are committed to giving it your best shot. There is just one small detail holding you back—you feel lost in your own kitchen. You may be stumped as to how to turn kamut, quinoa, tofu, and tempeh into tasty meals. All of this newness can seem terribly daunting. Fear not. This part of the change process can be an extraordinary adventure—one filled with amazing discoveries and wonderfully tantalizing flavors and textures. Embrace the challenge—experiment with these new foods, buy some interesting recipe books, take cooking classes, and do what it takes to make these new foods your trusted allies.

A number of concerns may arise as you embark on this quest. Will your efforts limit the range of foods you have to choose from? Will you have to shop at special stores? Will your grocery bill shoot through the roof? Won't all of this whole foods cooking be awfully time consuming? Will you need all kinds of expensive kitchen equipment? While such questions are understandable, it is reassuring to discover that although this way of eating is different and new for many of you, it offers every bit as much variety. While special stores can be helpful and fun to explore, most of what you will need is available from the supermarket. While food preparation does take time, you'll become more adept as you learn, and soon you can be just as efficient as ever in the kitchen. As for special equipment, there are a few trade-offs, but no huge changes. This chapter is one that is filled with practical support and tips to make your transition both enjoyable and entertaining.

WHAT TO BUY

Let's begin with your shopping list. What should you fill your freezer, refrigerator, and pantry with? Your shopping list must include basics for everyday cooking, as well as fresh foods that will need to be replaced on a weekly basis. It is helpful if you predetermine what your main meals will be for the week, so you can pick up all the necessary ingredients for your recipes. The list on the facing page provides a great start. It can be copied as is, or personalized to suit your needs.

WHERE TO BUY

When you look over your grocery list, the first thought that comes to mind may be where on earth you find such things. You will be surprised to learn that most of these items can be found in most supermarkets, and all are available in larger natural food stores. However, you may also wish to explore a number of other options, as many offer excellent value. You are likely to come across some interesting alternatives that are very close to home: some amazing little store that you never knew existed, an organic delivery service that brings fresh organic produce right to your door step.

Here are a few of the most popular choices.

Supermarkets   The large chains have come a long way in recent years, and many have expanded their organic produce departments, bulk food sections, ethnic options, and natural food sections. Conventional wisdom tells

BASIC SHOPPING LIST

GRAINS

___ Brown rice
___ Barley & millet
___ Kamut, spelt, wheat berries
___ Oat groats
___ Quinoa & other grains
___ Oatmeal & other hot cereals
___ Cold, whole grain cereals
___ Wheat germ
___ Flours (whole-wheat, unbleached, rye, other)
___ Pasta
___ Popcorn
___ Whole grain bread, buns, bagels
___ Whole grain crackers

BEANS, LENTILS & MEAT SUBSTITUTES

___ Dried legumes (garbanzos, navy, pinto & kidney beans, lentils, split peas)
___ Canned legumes (garbanzos, pinto, kidney, baked beans)
___ Frozen legumes (edamame-green soybeans)
___ Tofu, tempeh
___ Instant dried legume dishes (hummus, soups, casseroles, refried beans)
___ Meat substitutes, vegetarian patties, soy wieners, veggie slices, sausages
___ Prepared bean dishes (soups & chili)
___ Seitan (prepared gluten)
___ Soy nuts

NUTS, SEEDS, BUTTERS

___ Nut butters
___ Nuts (raw cashews, almonds, walnuts, pecans)
___ Seed butters (tahini)
___ Seeds (flax, pumpkin, sesame, sunflower)

VEGETABLES & FRUITS

___ Fresh greens (kale, collards, Chinese/napa cabbage, broccoli, lettuce)
___ Seasonal fresh vegetables
___ Garlic & onions
___ Seasonal fresh fruits
___ Frozen fruit
___ Frozen vegetables
___ Canned water-packed fruits
___ Canned tomatoes, tomato sauce, & other tomato products
___ Dried fruits (raisins, figs, apricots, dates, prunes, cranberries, currants, others)
___ Fruit and vegetable juices (fresh, frozen, bottled, canned & in tetra packs)

SOY & GRAIN BEVERAGES & RELATED PRODUCTS

___ Fortified soy & grain milks
___ Soy yogurt

DAIRY PRODUCTS & EGGS (IF USED)

___ Skim or low-fat milk
___ Reduced-fat cottage cheese
___ Very low-fat cheese
___ Low-fat yogurt
___ Eggs

SWEETENERS

___ Agave syrup barley malt, rice syrup, maple syrup, others
___ Dried sweeteners
___ Stevia
___ Blackstrap molasses
___ Low-sugar jams, conserves

BEVERAGES

___ Cereal grain beverages
___ Leaf & herbal teas
___ Organic coffee (if used)

FATS & OILS

___ Extra-virgin olive oil
___ Flaxseed oil
___ Mayonnaise or mayonnaise-like spread
___ Non-hydrogenated margarine
___ Nut oils (hazelnut, walnut)
___ Organic canola oil, high-oleic sunflower, safflower oils
___ Toasted sesame oil
___ Vegetable or lecithin spray

SEASONINGS, OTHER

___ Bragg Liquid Aminos
___ Vegetarian Support Formula Nutritional Yeast (Red Star)
___ Bottled sauces (teriyaki, barbeque, sweet & sour, other)
___ Cooking wine
___ Ketchup, mustard & relish
___ Lemon juice
___ Miso
___ Patak's or other curry paste
___ Pickles
___ Tamari or soy sauce
___ Seaweed (hijiki, wakame, nori, agar)
___ Vegetable broth powder & cubes, chicken-style seasoning
___ Vinegar (rice, wine, balsamic & apple cider vinegar)

HERBS & SPICES

___ Chili powder, hot chili peppers
___ Cinnamon, allspice, nutmeg, cloves, cardamom
___ Curry, cumin, turmeric
___ Dried herbs (oregano, basil, sage, savory, thyme)
___ Fresh gingerroot
___ Fresh herbs (parsley, basil)
___ Mixed seasonings (Spike)
___ Mustard, powdered
___ Salt & pepper

us to shop in the perimeter isles, as these contain the least processed foods. However, the perimeter contains a great deal of high-fat, high-cholesterol animal products, such as meat and cheese, so you need to go a step beyond the perimeter rule in your thinking. Begin in the produce section. In many stores, this is also where the tofu and veggie "meats" are kept. Many of the most healthful foods are in the bulk section, including whole grains, nuts, seeds, and legumes. Don't forget the natural food section for soymilk and any packaged foods, such as cereal or crackers.

Natural Food Stores   Large natural food stores are becoming more popular and more accessible. Although some "health food" stores seem to be supplement stores with very few food items, many specialize in vegetarian and organic foods. They carry a wide assortment of beans, less-common whole grains, and other products (pasta, for instance) made with whole grain flours such as quinoa, spelt, and kamut. On the shelves and in coolers and freezers are convenience foods without hydrogenated vegetable oils, food colors, artificial flavors, preservatives, or other additives. These stores also often carry organic produce, whole grain baked goods, tofu, soymilk, and other nondairy milks, refrigerated nuts, nut butters, and wholesome snacks such as fat-free tortilla chips and fruit bars. Many also carry organic animal products such as milk and eggs. For health-conscious consumers, locating a good natural food store can be like finding a treasure chest.

Farmers' Markets/Direct Purchase from Farmers   If you live in an area surrounded by farms, you will also likely find farmers' markets. Most include a number of venders who grow and sell organic produce. Farmers' markets generally offer very competitive prices and bulk sales. Prices are often at least 30 percent less than what's charged in supermarkets. Most of the produce is locally grown and freshly picked. Many markets include items that are not commonly available at supermarkets—unusual greens such as purslane, collards, and chard, and uncommon vegetables such as purple potatoes, Jerusalem artichokes, and salad turnips. Sometimes local farmers also sell directly to consumers. Some sell prepicked fruits and vegetables, while others offer a "U-pick" option for reduced prices. Another interesting possibility is participating in a CSA—community-supported agriculture project—where you purchase shares in the yield of a cooperative garden, with payment coming back in the form of a variety of produce throughout the growing season.

Organic Delivery Services   Many communities offer incredible organic delivery services that provide healthful, high-quality, organically grown fruits and vegetables in a fun and convenient way. These services deliver a box of fresh, often locally grown, produce to your front door. Many such services allow custom orders (you select the items you want each week), and some offer additional items such as organic breads, fresh-pressed oils, salad dressings, and apple cider. Buying from such a service not only supports a small local business, but it supports many organic farmers in your area and elsewhere.

Ethnic Shops   Most larger towns and cities feature a unique mix of ethnic food stores. These stores provide a wide range of wonderful food options, and an interesting lesson about the food traditions of other cultures. Asian stores carry a wonderful selection of tofu, fresh greens, seaweeds, seitan (gluten), edamame, and Asian sauces. Many of these are available at far lower prices than what you can find elsewhere. Middle-Eastern stores supply high-quality olive oil, olives, and tahini, as well as ready-made falafel, tabouli, and fresh pita bread. East Indian stores carry a variety of flours, curry pastes, beans, grains, and spice mixes. Don't hesitate to ask questions; the proprietors are generally very happy to offer advice!

Buying Clubs   Buying clubs are groups of friends, relatives, neighbors, or colleagues that get together to place bulk food orders from wholesalers. They usually include at least three or four people or families, as most wholesalers require minimum orders of several hundred dollars. It is easy to find the names of wholesalers—simply look them up in the phone book or ask your natural food store who they might suggest you deal with. The discount may be almost as much as what is given to stores. Foods come in large quantities, such as a case or a 25-pound bag (11.4 kg). Buying from a wholesaler means organizing the orders, pickups, and division of food, but it can save a lot of time and money in the long run. You often end up with large enough supplies to last a long time. A weigh scale is very important in helping to divide up the goods.

FOOD LABELS: GETTING PAST THE CLAIMS

No cholesterol, low-fat, all-natural...these kinds of claims are front and center of many food labels. However, this is not where our most telling nutrition information lies. Instead, it is tucked away on the sides or back of the container in the nutrition facts and ingredient list. A food label can be an awesome ally if you know how to use it. It pays to invest a little time into understanding label lingo and what a food manufacturer can do with it. Regulations from the Food and Drug Administration (FDA) and the Food Safety and Inspection Service (FSIS) of the United States Department of Agriculture (USDA) ensure that almost every packaged food comes with nutrition labeling. This labeling includes two essential components: the nutrition panel and ingredient list; and two optional components: nutrient content descriptors and health claims.

The Nutrition Panel

The nutrition panel appears under the title "Nutrition Facts." This panel provides most of the details you will require regarding the nutritional contents of a food. Serving sizes are uniform across all product lines so that nutrients in similar food items can be easily compared. Nutrition information is expressed as a percent of a dietary reference value called the "Daily Value" (DV). The DVs are based on the nutritional needs of an individual consuming a 2,000-calorie diet. Most panels include the following information per serving of the food: calories, calories from fat, total fat, saturated fat, cholesterol, sodium, total carbohydrate, fiber, sugar, and protein, plus the percent of the DVs for all but sugar and protein. Daily Values for vitamin A, vitamin C, calcium, and iron are also listed, while those of other vitamins and minerals need only be provided when a claim is made about them on the label.

The Ingredient List

A full list of ingredients must appear on all packaged processed foods, including standardized foods such as bread and jelly which were previously exempt. New regulations provide for a more thorough description of ingredients such as food colors and protein hydrolysates (which must identify their source to assist people with allergies). Foods claiming to be "nondairy" (i.e., nondairy creamer) must identify caseinate as a milk derivative in the ingredient statement.

Ingredients are listed according to weight, with the ingredient present in the largest amount listed first. This list can often answer questions regarding nutrition claims or nutrition information. For example, a package of commercial cookies may claim to be low in saturated fat. This sounds good, but if you examine the ingredient list, you see enriched flour (white flour) and vegetable oil shortening as the first two ingredients. As you may recall from chapter 3, shortening contains trans fatty acids, which are classified as monounsaturated fats, but are even more damaging than saturated fats. To help ensure that the product you are buying is everything it's cracked up to be, look for the following.

✓ Whole grain flour as the principle grain in the product (even multigrain products often have "enriched flour" or "wheat flour" as a first ingredient—both are refined white flours).

✓ The absence of shortening, lard, hydrogenated, or partially-hydrogenated vegetable oil, or other hard fats.

✓ Sweeteners that provide some nutritional value (i.e., concentrated fruit juices, dried fruits, or blackstrap molasses).

✓ An ingredient list with words you recognize. Some unfamiliar words are harmless everyday items (e.g., sodium bicarbonate is baking soda), but a readable list provides some assurance that the product is wholesome.

Nutrient Content Descriptors

Manufacturers are permitted to use terms that describe the nutrient content of a product in accordance with the new FDA regulations. These regulations ensure that whenever a description is used, it means the same thing on all food labels. For example, when a label states a product is "low-fat, low-cholesterol," it must contain less than 3 grams of fat, 20 mg cholesterol, and 2 grams saturated fat per serving.

Food producers can use nutrient content descriptions in ways that are confusing to consumers. For example, the label on a jar of peanut butter may read "cholesterol-free," leading people to believe that other brands of peanut butter are high in cholesterol. In fact, no peanut butter (or any other plant food) contains cholesterol.

Health Claims

Claims that link a nutrient or food to health or disease are permitted under certain circumstances. There are twelve diet and disease relationships for which claims are allowed. They include

- Calcium and osteoporosis
- Fat and cancer
- Saturated fat and cholesterol and coronary heart disease (CHD)
- Fiber-containing grain products, fruits, and vegetables and cancer
- Fruits, vegetables, and grain products that contain fiber and risk of CHD
- Sodium and hypertension (high blood pressure)
- Fruits and vegetables and cancer
- Folic acid and neural tube defects
- Dietary sugar alcohols and dental caries (cavities)
- Soluble fiber from certain foods, such as whole oats and psyllium seed husk, and CHD

- Soy protein and CHD
- Plant sterols and plant stanol esters and CHD

Any product making a claim about the above relationships must provide a specified amount of the nutrient in question or, as in the case of fat and cholesterol, must not exceed the specified amount.

For further information, the USDA has a more detailed description of food labels at http://www.cfsan.fda.gov/~dms/fdnewlab.html

SAFE STORAGE

I t is a good feeling to load up on the kinds of foods that you know will support and protect your health, but an awful disappointment if the food rapidly deteriorates or becomes rancid. Proper storage can make all the difference when it comes to maintaining the quality of the food you purchase. In storing food, there are three primary objectives.

1. To keep food fresh and appealing
2. To prevent spoilage, mold, rancidity, or infestations of bugs
3. To maximize nutrient retention

Appropriate food storage is especially important when your diet is based on unrefined foods. While these foods are highly nourishing to people, they are also feasts for bugs. On the other hand, foods that have been stripped of their nutrient value, such as white sugar and white flour, are far less interesting to such critters.

Grains

Nature does a fine job of protecting whole grains from becoming damaged by giving them a hard outer coat. As soon as we break this coat, grains can deteriorate much more quickly.

Storage Guidelines

Intact whole grains (wheat, kamut, and spelt berries, millet, quinoa, oat groats, and others)—Keep in tightly covered containers in a cool, dry place for up to two years.

Whole grain flour—Keep in tightly covered containers in a cool, dry place for up to two months, but it is best stored in the refrigerator where it will last for up to three to four months.

Wheat germ—Store in a covered container or plastic bag in the refrigerator or freezer.

Legumes and Legume-Based Products

Dried beans keep very well, however products made with beans must be more carefully stored.

Storage Guidelines

Dried beans—Store in a cool, dry place in a tightly covered container for up to a year or more. Dry beans will keep almost indefinitely; however, as they get older, they become harder to digest. It is best to buy beans in relatively small quantities and cook them within a few months.

Textured soy protein and soy protein powders—Store up to a year or more in a tightly covered container in a cool, dry place. Unflavored textured soy may keep for several years in a cool, dry place.

Tofu—Store in the refrigerator and use by the "best before" date. Once opened, store in a covered container and immerse with water. Use within a few days.

Tempeh—Keep for several days in the refrigerator, or in the freezer for longer-term storage.

Veggie burgers, wieners, deli slices, and other veggie "meats"—Store in the refrigerator and use by the "best before" date. Once opened, use within a few days. Freeze for longer-term storage.

Soymilk—Tetra packs: Store in a cool, dry place and use by the "best before" date. Once opened, store in the refrigerator and use within a week. Fresh: Store in the refrigerator and use by the "best before" date.

Nuts, Seeds, and Their Butters

Nuts and seeds come packaged by nature to protect the valuable contents within their shells. Once the shell is broken, these high-fat nutrition power-houses deteriorate quickly.

Storage Guidelines

Whole nuts in the shell and whole seeds—Store for up to a year in a cool, dry place.

Shelled nuts and ground seeds—Store in an airtight container in the refrigerator for up to four months or in the freezer for up to a year. Walnuts are best kept in the freezer due to their high omega-3 content. Walnuts that are not stored properly quickly become bitter. Other shelled nuts can be stored in a cool, dry place (unrefrigerated), in containers with lids, for up to two months (although refrigeration is preferable).

Ground flaxseeds—Store in the refrigerator up to two months, or in the freezer up to six months.

Nut and seed butters—Store for six to nine months if unopened. Once opened, store in the refrigerator for up to four months.

Fresh Fruits and Vegetables

Fresh fruits and vegetables are very perishable and must handled with care.

Storage Guidelines

Most fresh fruits—Ripen at room temperature and then refrigerate until ready to use (refrigeration stops further ripening) or for up to two weeks.

Most fresh vegetables—Refrigerate immediately after purchase and use within a week. As tomatoes are botanically a fruit, they are best ripened and eaten at room temperature, but can be refrigerated after ripening. Lettuce and other greens keep well in plastic containers with tight-fitting lids. You can get specially manufactured produce storage bags that do a wonderful job of extending the freshness of your produce in the refrigerator.

Potatoes, sweet potatoes, onions, garlic, squash—Store in a dark, cool, dry place for up to a few weeks.

Other Items

Vegetable oils—Refined oils can be stored in a cool, dark place for up to a year, unopened. Once opened, they are best used within two months. If you purchase larger portions than you can use in this time, it is best to refrigerate the oil. Unrefined oils are more perishable. Oils rich in omega-3 fatty acids (flaxseed, hempseed and walnut oils) must be kept refrigerated. Use within two months. Oils are damaged by light, heat, and oxygen, so it is best to minimize their exposure to these elements.

Animal products—Dairy products and eggs must be refrigerated, and other animal products must be refrigerated or frozen.

Dry baker's yeast—If unopened, store at room temperature in a cool, dry place until its expiration date. Once opened, keep airtight and refrigerated.

Nutritional yeast—Store in a cool, dry place; however, to prevent infestation by insects, store larger quantities in the freezer, keeping out only as much as would be used up in about a month.

Canned goods—Store canned foods for up to one year. Although the product is generally safe after this time, the color, flavor, texture, and nutritive value may deteriorate. Store contents of an opened can in a clean, covered container, and refrigerate for up to one week.

Jarred goods—Unopened salad dressings, jams, jellies, liquid sugars, soup mixes, ketchup, and chili sauce keep up to one year.

Organizing Pantry Storage

When you begin to use a wide variety of beans and grains, you may end up with so many plastic bags of goods that you can never find what you are looking for. It can be a most frustrating experience when trying to prepare a recipe efficiently. A little organization will make food preparation a lot less stressful. Keep grains, beans, dried fruits, seeds, chocolate chips, coconut, and other bulk dry goods in mason jars. Buy about three-dozen wide-mouth canning jars, label them, and arrange the filled jars on an open shelf or in the pantry. Bulkier items such as flour can be kept in larger canisters, plastic buckets with tight-fitting lids, or larger jars.

ESSENTIAL EQUIPMENT

hile you can manage with very few extras in the kitchen, having a few high-quality tools allows you to get your cooking done with greater efficiency. The following basics are highly recommended.

Three good-quality knives. The items that will most increase your enjoyment and efficiency in the kitchen are a large French knife (chef's knife), a small paring knife, and a bread knife with a serrated edge.

Cutting board. Wooden boards are definitely the best for cutting, although they are more difficult to clean than plastic or glass boards.

Mixing bowls. You will need at least three glass or stainless steel bowls of varying sizes. Deep, narrow bowls are especially handy.

Nonstick skillet. Invest in high quality cookware, if you can. Skillets should have good conducting ability and disperse heat evenly.

Two pots. As a minimum, get a large pot for soup or pasta and a smaller pot for cooked cereal, sauces, or steamed vegetables.

Stainless steel basket steamer. This inexpensive gadget fits into almost any size pot and is used to steam vegetables or veggie wieners.

Blender. Blenders are extremely useful for pureeing dressings, soups, shakes, and smoothies.

Strainer. This is helpful for draining liquid from cooked pasta, vegetables, potatoes, and legumes.

Handheld tools. Be sure to have measuring cups and spoons, a wooden spoon, food grater, can opener, vegetable peeler, flipper, rubber spatula, spring-loaded tongs, and perhaps a whisk.

Food processor. While not essential, a food processor is useful for making hummus, nut and seed butter, pâtés, and thick spreads.

Juicer. This can be a fancy machine or a simple stainless steel hand juicer. Look for one with two parts: the top part where the fruit is held, and the bottom part that holds the juice.

TRANSFORMING TRADITIONAL FAVORITES

T he switch to a whole foods, plant-based diet does not necessarily mean giving up all your favorite dishes. Instead, you can transform many of these dishes to more nutritious versions of former favorites. Table 11.1 provides workable substitutions for most recipes. Get creative and turn fat and cholesterol-laden fare into high-fiber, healthful dishes.

TABLE 11.1 | Instead of Meat, Egg, or Dairy: Substitution Basics

Instead of 1 cup (250 mL) meat or chicken stock, choose:

1 cup (250 mL) liquid vegetable stock (in tetra packs or made from vegetable stock cubes or powder); Bragg Liquid Aminos, tamari, or miso mixed with water (to taste)

Instead of 1 serving meat or chicken, choose:

• Equal weight or volume of veggie "meat," plain, herbed, or marinated tofu, tempeh, beans, gluten (seitan), gluten-based "meats" from Asian restaurants
• Equal volume of portobello mushrooms

Instead of 1 cup (250 mL) ground beef, choose:

• Equal weight or volume of vegetarian "ground round" (frozen or fresh)
• ½ cup (125 mL) dry textured soy protein, covered with boiling stock or water, stirred, and soaked for ten minutes

Instead of 1 burger patty or wiener, choose:

1 veggie burger or 1 veggie wiener (there are numerous varieties to choose from)

Instead of scrambled eggs, choose:

Scrambled Tofu (see recipe on page 206)

Instead of eggs in savory dishes, choose:

This can be tricky, but a combination of tofu and ground nuts can work well, especially in veggie burgers, loaves, or veggie roasts; replace 2 eggs with ¼ cup (60 mL) of tofu and 2 Tbsp. (30 mL) of ground nuts or sunflower seeds

Instead of eggs in baked goods, choose (per egg):

- 1 Tbsp. (15 mL) ground flaxseed mixed with 3 Tbsp. (45 mL) water
- 2–4 Tbsp. (30–60 mL) soft tofu
- ¼ cup (60 mL) mashed, very ripe banana
- 1 tsp. (5 mL) starch-based egg substitute (powdered products that replace eggs in baking)
- ⅛ tsp. (0.6 mL) baking powder, added to dry ingredients, provides the leavening action of 1 egg or egg white

Instead of 1 cup (250 mL) whole cow's milk, choose:

1 cup (250 mL) fortified soymilk, rice milk, or skim milk

Instead of 1 cup (250 mL) whole buttermilk, choose:

1 cup (250 mL) soymilk plus 2 tsp. (10 mL) lemon juice or vinegar, or skim buttermilk

Instead of 1 cup (250 mL) full-fat yogurt, choose:

1 cup (250 mL) soy yogurt or nonfat yogurt

Instead of 1 oz. (28 g) cheese, choose:

1 oz. (28 g) very low-fat or nonfat cheese, or 1 oz. (28 g) soy cheese (made without hydrogenated fat)

Instead of 1 cup (250 mL) cottage cheese or ricotta cheese (in recipes), choose:

1 cup (250 mL) drained, mashed tofu (medium firm for cottage cheese and firm for ricotta cheese)

Instead of 1½ cups (375 mL) whipping cream, choose:

12 oz. (340 g) package firm silken tofu, ¼ cup (60 mL) maple syrup, 1 Tbsp. (15 mL) lemon juice, and 1 tsp. (5 mL) vanilla, blended

Instead of butter, choose:

Olive oil or nonhydrogenated margarine (total fat does not change, however type of fat improves)

MAKING THE TRANSITION TO A PLANT-BASED DIET

A mong the best ways of ensuring delicious and nutritious meals is to begin with fresh, high-quality ingredients. Fresh herbs and garlic, a squeeze of lemon, and a touch of extra-virgin olive oil can turn a ho-hum dish into a something special. Choose a variety of colors and textures in the foods you prepare. Take the time to make meals look appealing.

Whether it's breakfast, lunch, dinner, or snacks, you'll want your food to be interesting, tasty, and nutritious. Don't fall into the rut of eating the same foods day in and day out. Experiment with all kinds of flavors, including those with which you aren't so familiar. The following pages will provide you with a host of practical suggestions for making the most of your meals.

Breakfast Basics

Most people don't set aside much time for their morning meal, if they bother with it at all. Unfortunately, skipping breakfast robs people of a number of important advantages. Breakfast eaters have better concentration, are more efficient workers, are more creative, and have a better sense of well-being. Not surprisingly, they live longer too.

The challenge is to make breakfast a priority in your life. You'll need to allow at least fifteen minutes to avoid being too rushed with your meal.

A healthful breakfast provides about a quarter of your daily nutrient needs and a generous portion of fiber and phytochemicals. By selecting a variety of foods from the plant-based food guide on pages 100-109, it's hard to go wrong. Breakfast is probably the easiest meal for incorporating intact whole grains. (See the recipe on page 203. While this combination of grains may be new to you, if you like hot cereals, you will love this one.) If using processed breads and cereals, select those made with only whole grains. Include a good source of vitamin C and other antioxidant nutrients. Fresh fruits are great choices. Be sure to include a good source of protein such as tofu, soymilk, veggie "meats," nuts, or nut butters. Nonfat cheese, nonfat yogurt, and eggs (in moderation) can also be used, if desired.

Reducing intake of eggs and high-fat dairy products is getting easier all the time. Nondairy beverages made from soy, tofu, nuts, and rice can be used as a direct substitute for cow's milk on cereal and in most recipes. Select varieties that are fortified with calcium, vitamin D, and vitamin B_{12}.

The following breakfast suggestions are all fast, nutritious, and delicious.

- Scrambled tofu or leftover savory beans served with cornbread or whole grain muffins and fresh orange or grapefruit sections
- Hot cereal using a combination of grains and spices (top it off with some sliced fruit, wheat germ, nuts, or ground flaxseed and soymilk or skim milk)
- Ready-to-eat muesli with almonds, berries, and soymilk
- Multigrain toast with tahini or almond butter and blackstrap molasses plus fresh fruit salad
- Whole grain pancakes, waffles, or French toast served with veggie ham or sausages, topped with fresh fruit or fruit sauce

Let's Do Lunch

Whether you take a brown bag for lunch, dine out, or eat at home, lunch meals can be fast, easy, and very enjoyable.

Business or Restaurant Lunch

With the tremendous boom of interest in health, it has become much easier to find appealing, plant-based meals in restaurants. Among your very best options are ethnic restaurants, as you will recall from chapter 8. Salads, soups, veggie stir-fries, and bean dishes are all great options. Even fast-food restaurants generally offer veggie burgers and salads.

Bag Lunches

The key to enticing, plant-based bag lunches is to get creative. Free yourself from the notion that lunch must come between two slices of bread. Carry soup, stew, or chili in a thermos. Bring a marinated salad, some rice and vegetable stir-fry, or lettuce wraps. Even sandwiches can be innovative and interesting. Start with rice wrappers, whole grain pita bread, heavy rye bread, or flaxseed bagels. Fill them with hummus and sprouts; thin slices of flavored tofu, tomato slices, and lettuce; veggie burgers, onions, and dill pickles; or tofu salad, olives, and red peppers.

House Specials

You have the greatest flexibility when eating at home. Lunch is a great time to include legumes. Add them to a hearty vegetable soup or salad. When making these items, prepare enough for several meals. Soups generally freeze very well. Leftovers also serve as good lunch meals, especially stews and other one-pot dishes. Be sure to include at least one vegetable with this meal.

What's for Dinner?

How do we transform a meal that is traditionally centered around meat to being a delicious plant-based alternative? That presents a bit of a challenge for the new vegetarian. To make dinner meals both simple and enjoyable, here are a couple of options.

- *Modify traditional style meals.* Simply replace the meat in traditional meals with beans, tofu, tempeh, seitan (gluten), veggie burgers or wieners, veggie ground round, nuts, or textured vegetable protein. You can still have all your favorite trimmings like mashed potatoes and gravy, corn on the cob, dressing, and vegetables.

- *Go ethnic.* Borrow some ideas from the cultures that rarely use meat or use it in very small quantities. Try Mexican, Lebanese, East Indian, Chinese, or African dishes. When you first begin preparing vegetarian dinners, you may find it easiest to make traditional meals most of the time, gradually incorporating ethnic foods into your repertoire. Before you know it, you'll be whipping up interesting dishes from around the world. Of course, if you have the advantage of growing up in a culture that uses very little meat, your task will be that much easier.

If you're concerned about the time it takes to cook plant-based meals, relax. They needn't take longer to prepare than meals with meat.

Fixing Fast Dinners

Whether you like to prepare things from scratch or prefer to rely on ready-made convenience foods, there are many things that you can do to make the whole process more efficient.

- Prepare meals in advance. When you plan ahead, you can walk in the house at 6:00 P.M. to a nice, hot meal just waiting in the crock-pot. It means soaking beans ahead of time and allowing time to cut up vegetables in the morning. Needless to say, it's well worth the effort.

■ Cook batches of at least double what you or your family can eat in one meal. Making double or triple batches means that you'll be able to enjoy an evening or weekend off somewhere down the road. You can save leftovers for the next day or freeze a batch for later use. Cook grains and beans in large quantities too. Package them in meal-sized portions and freeze, or plan a couple of different dishes using them as a base. For example, you may serve a vegetable/cashew stir-fry with brown rice for supper one day, then some curried tofu with the leftover rice a day or two later.

■ Stock your pantry and freezer well. If you haven't tried any of the plant-based convenience foods that are on the market, you're in for a treat. With the tremendous variety of these products, you can have a meal ready in minutes. Keep a variety of the following foods on hand.

Canned lentils and beans. Add to soups, spaghetti sauces, chili, or casseroles. Firmer beans such as garbanzos can be thrown into a stir-fry. Freeze-dried beans (such as freeze-dried refried beans or bean soups) are particularly useful for backpacking or camping.

Tofu. A wonderful convenience food, tofu can be made into a meal in a matter of minutes. It can be stir-fried, baked, scrambled, added to soups, stews, burritos, or made into patties, loaves, or roasts. Tofu can be frozen and thawed to obtain a pleasant, chewy consistency.

Quick whole grains. Quick-cooking wild or brown rice and pastas are now available in most stores. Bulgar wheat, whole grain couscous, millet, and quinoa all can be prepared in less than thirty minutes.

Wheat gluten products (seitan). The concentrated protein in wheat flour is kneaded, seasoned, and cooked to produce seitan or "wheat meat." Its chewy texture often resembles beef or chicken, making it great in stews, soups, and casseroles.

Frozen foods. There are wonderful discoveries to be made in the frozen section of health food stores and supermarkets. In addition to vegetables and legumes, you'll find veggie "meats," tempeh, complete, nutritious entrees, and whole-wheat bread dough.

Getting Familiar with Beans and Grains

The preparation of wonderful new recipes (including those in the next chapter) can be a tremendously rewarding experience. This can be the foundation of many pleasant evenings shared with friends or family members. If you are new to the world of whole plant foods, you may need to incorporate a few new tricks into your kitchen routine, especially where less familiar foods are concerned. Many wonderful tips are sprinkled throughout the recipe section. Two of the primary stumbling blocks for beginners to whole foods diets are legumes and whole grains. The following information will help provide the basics of preparing these wonderfully versatile foods.

Cooking Legumes

Some legumes are small and do not need presoaking before cooking. These include lentils, mung beans, and split peas. However, if you do have time to presoak them, it will speed up cooking time and increase mineral availability. For every cup of these small legumes, use 3 cups (750 mL) of water. Cooking time varies from about 25 minutes to an hour for unsoaked lentils, mung beans, and split peas.

Larger dried beans (all other legumes) must be presoaked before cooking. This includes kidney, adzuki, lima, pinto, garbanzo, navy, white, and black beans, and many others. To cook these beans, first sort through them to remove any small stones and bad beans, and soak overnight for 6 hours or more in at least triple the volume of water. The soaking time can be shortened by bringing the beans to a boil, then removing from them from the heat and soaking for 1 hour. Discard the liquid, rinse, cover with fresh water, and cook for the recommended time or until tender. Discard the water and rinse the beans thoroughly. Cover the beans with about 3 inches of fresh, unsalted water, and boil vigorously for 1 minute. Cover and simmer for 1 to 3 hours. Very hard water (high in minerals) can increase bean cooking time. Beans can also be cooked all day or overnight in a slow cooker. For every cup (250 mL) of soaked beans, add 3 cups (750 mL) of fresh water.

Beans cook much faster in a pressure cooker. You can also sprout your dried beans for two to three days before cooking to shorten the cooking time. Be sure to cook beans until they are soft enough to press between your tongue and the roof of your mouth. Our digestive systems can't handle crunchy beans.

PRACTICAL POINTER

We all know that eating beans can keep us regular. Unfortunately, they can also cause the uncomfortable and embarrassing problem of gas. To reduce gas production from beans, soak and rinse them three to five times over at least a day or two. This will enable you to enjoy generous helpings of beans without the side effects.

Cooking Grains

Grains should generally be rinsed in a colander before cooking. In a pot with a lid, combine the grains with the measured amount of water, bring to a boil, cover, reduce the heat, and simmer for the recommended time. If you have hard water, cooking time will be longer.

Large intact grains (such as kamut, spelt, wheat or rye berries, barley, and oat groats)—Use 1 cup (250 mL) rinsed grains and 3 cups (750 mL) water. Cook 40 to 50 minutes for barley and about 1 hour for other grains.

Smaller grains or cut grains (such as millet, quinoa, amaranth, cracked wheat, brown rice, and buckwheat) — Use 1 cup (250 mL) rinsed grains and 2 cups (500 mL) of water for rice, cracked wheat, amaranth, and quinoa and 2½ cups (625 mL) water for others. All these grains cook in 20 to 30 minutes, except rice, which takes about 45 minutes. Bulgur does not need to be cooked, just soaked in boiling water.

Smart Snacks

For many people with diabetes, snacks are an important part of daily food intake. Often in our society, snacks are associated with junk food such as potato chips and doughnuts, thus snacking is sometimes viewed negatively. When you choose snacks wisely, they can have a very positive impact on your overall nutrient intake and absorption. The following tips will help to make your selections a snap:

✓ Select your snacks from the plant-based food guide. If it's not part of the guide, then chances are it's not a good choice.

✓ Keep nutritious choices handy. You tend to eat whatever is most convenient when you're hungry. If only nutritious choices are available, that's what you'll choose.

✓ Be especially selective when away from home. Stop at a produce place for fresh fruit, at a deli for a marinated salad, or a natural food store for some soy nuts and yogurt.

✓ Bring food from home. When you know healthful options will be hard to come by, this is your best bet.

✓ Include foods from food groups that you tend to fall short on. For example, if you seem to fall short on legume choices, opt for flavored tofu, pea or black bean soup, or crackers with deli slices.

The following snacks will ensure that your snack choices make a real contribution to your nutrient needs, and to your blood sugar control.

- Raw vegetables with a tofu, yogurt, or bean-based dip
- Fresh fruit salad topped with yogurt
- Celery stuffed with nut butter
- Pea soup and crackers
- Marinated vegetable and bean salad
- Whole grain pudding with fruit sauce
- Rye crisps or rice cakes with deli slices and pickles
- Edamame (soybeans in the shell cooked in salted water)
- Homemade whole grain muffin with almond butter
- Raw vegetables with tofu or yogurt dip
- Trail mix or nut mixes
- Whole grain crackers and antipasto
- Lettuce wraps made with baked or flavored tofu and shredded vegetables
- Baked tortilla chips, refried beans, and salsa
- Hummus and pita bread
- Tabouli salad with garbanzo beans
- Cold cereal with berries and soymilk
- Soynuts and fresh fruit
- Whole grain bagel half with nonfat cheese and tomato slices
- Popcorn sprayed with Bragg Liquid Aminos and flax oil, and sprinkled with nutritional yeast

CHAPTER 12

Recipes for Defeating Diabetes

n this chapter, we will take you from breakfast through to dinner and snacks, with some fabulous recipes. Many of these are sure to become staples in your home. Enjoy!

WHOLE GRAIN WAFFLES

Serves 5 (1 waffle per serving)

⅓ cup (85 mL) cornmeal

⅔ cup (165 mL) whole-wheat flour

½ cup (125 mL) oat flour

½ cup (125 mL) rice flour

3 tablespoons (45 mL) ground flaxseed*

2 teaspoons (10 mL) baking powder

¼ teaspoon (1.2 mL) salt

2 tablespoons (30 mL) canola oil

⅔ cup (165 mL) water

1½ cups (375 mL) soymilk or nonfat milk

Preheat waffle iron.

In a medium mixing bowl, combine the cornmeal, flours, flaxseed, baking powder, and salt. Make a well in the middle of the dry ingredients and add the oil, water, and soymilk or milk. Stir just until blended. Batter should be slightly lumpy.

Ladle batter onto waffle iron. Cook until golden brown. If desired, serve waffles topped with yogurt and chopped fruit or berries.

*To grind flaxseed, place in an electric mill, such as the type used to grind coffee beans, and pulse until finely ground, or crush using a heavy mortar and pestle.

See glossary:

Canola oil

Flaxseed

Oat flour

Rice flour

Soymilk

1 SERVING = 1 WAFFLE = 2 GRAINS + 1 NUT/SEED

PER WAFFLE	total fat-10 g	sodium-266 mg	iron-2.5 mg
calories-264	(saturated fat-1 g)	potassium-284 mg	calcium-161 mg
protein-8 g	fiber-5.8 g	vitamin A-7 RE	phosphorus-403 mg
carbohydrates-38 g	cholesterol-0 mg	vitamin C-0 mg	

Rich source of omega-3 fatty acids (providing at least 1 g per serving)

WHOLE GRAIN BREAKFAST CEREAL

Serves 8 (1 cup/250 mL per serving)

Serve the cereal with soymilk and fresh berries or dried fruit.
Refrigerate the leftovers to enjoy for several mornings.

1 cup (250 mL) barley
1 cup (250 mL) millet
1 cup (250 mL) oat groats
7 cups (1¾ L) water

Rinse and soak the barley, millet, and oat groats overnight in the water.

In the morning, bring the grains to a boil in a large saucepan, then lower the heat to a simmer and cook covered for 40 to 50 minutes, or until tender and the water has been absorbed, stirring occasionally. Add more water if the cereal sticks to the pan.

TIP: Make the cereal the night before in a crock pot. Eliminate the soaking step and reduce the amount of water based on crock pot manufacturer's recommendations.

See glossary:

Barley
Millet
Oat groats

1 SERVING = 1 CUP/250 mL = 3 GRAINS			
PER SERVING	total fat-3 g	sodium-4 mg	iron-2.3 mg
calories-260	(saturated fat-1 g)	potassium-189 mg	calcium-20 mg
protein-7 g	fiber-5.7 g	vitamin A-1 RE	phosphorus-209 mg
carbohydrates-53 g	cholesterol-0 mg	vitamin C-0 mg	

ﬔRENCH TOAST

Serves 6 (1 slice per serving)

¼ cup (60 mL) rolled oats
⅓ cup (85 mL) raw cashews
1 cup (250 mL) soymilk or nonfat milk
⅛ teaspoon (0.6 mL) vanilla extract
⅛ teaspoon (0.6 mL) cinnamon
⅛ teaspoon (0.6 mL) salt (optional)
6 slices whole-wheat bread

Place oats, cashews, soymilk or milk, vanilla, cinnamon, and salt, if using, in food processor or blender and process until blended. Pour batter into a shallow baking dish. Dip the bread slices in the batter to coat both sides.

Preheat a large skillet over medium heat.

Cook the battered bread over medium heat, turning once, until golden brown. If desired, serve with yogurt and fruit.

See glossary:

Oats, rolled
Soymilk

1 SERVING = 1 SLICE = 1 GRAIN + ½ NUT/SEED			
PER SLICE	total fat-6 g	sodium-106 mg	iron-1.6 mg
calories-121	(saturated fat-1 g)	potassium-173 mg	calcium-7 mg
protein-5 g	fiber-3.1 g	vitamin A-2 RE	phosphorus-126 mg
carbohydrates-14 g	cholesterol-0 mg	vitamin C-0 mg	

MORNING MUESLI

Serves 4 (²/₃ cup/165 mL per serving)

½ cup (125 mL) oat bran
1 cup (250 mL) rolled oats
1¼ cups (310 mL) water
1 cup (250 mL) soymilk or nonfat milk
¼ cup (60 mL) sunflower seeds
¼ cup (60 mL) raisins
¼ cup (60 mL) chopped walnuts
1 apple, grated

The night before, mix all of the ingredients together in a medium bowl. Refrigerate overnight, covered.

Serve the muesli in the morning, with yogurt and sliced fresh fruit or berries, if desired.

See glossary:

Oat bran
Oats, rolled
Soymilk

1 SERVING = ²/₃ CUP/165 mL = 2 GRAINS + ½ FRUIT + ½ NUT/SEED			
PER SERVING	total fat-12 g	sodium-12 mg	iron-2.4 mg
calories-249	(saturated fat-1 g)	potassium-377 mg	calcium-36 mg
protein-9 g	fiber-6 g	vitamin A-7 RE	phosphorus-230 mg
carbohydrates-31 g	cholesterol-0 mg	vitamin C-3 mg	

SCRAMBLED TOFU

Serves 4 (¹/₂ cup/125 mL per serving)

2 cloves garlic, minced
¹/₂ cup (125 mL) red or green bell pepper, seeded, chopped
¹/₂ cup (125 mL) chopped onion
¹/₂ teaspoon (2.5 mL) canola or extra-virgin olive oil
1 pound (453 g) firm tofu, crumbled
1 tablespoon (15 mL) tamari
¹/₄ teaspoon (1.2 mL) turmeric
2 tablespoons (30 mL) nutritional yeast flakes

In a medium skillet, sauté the garlic, bell pepper, and onion in the oil over medium heat about 5 minutes, or until soft. Add the tofu, tamari, and turmeric, and heat, stirring occasionally, until the excess moisture cooks away and the tofu is somewhat dry. Stir in the yeast and remove from the heat.

See glossary:

Canola oil
Extra-virgin olive oil
Nutritional yeast flakes
Tamari
Tofu
Turmeric

1 SERVING = ¹/₂ CUP/125 mL = 1¹/₂ LEGUMES

PER SERVING:	total fat-11 g	sodium-269 mg	iron-12.2 mg
calories-194	(saturated fat-1 g)	potassium-406 mg	calcium-241 mg
protein-21 g	fiber-3.2 g	vitamin A-25 RE	phosphorus-273 mg
carbohydrates-9 g	cholesterol-0 mg	vitamin C-10 mg	

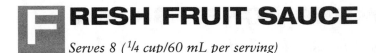RESH FRUIT SAUCE

Serves 8 (¹⁄₄ cup/60 mL per serving)

While your pancakes, waffles, or French toast cook,
prepare this simple sauce. Serve immediately;
because of the fresh bananas, it doesn't store well.

¹⁄₄ cup (60 mL) water
¹⁄₄ cup (60 mL) raisins
Juice of 1 lemon
1¹⁄₂ cups (375 mL) berries, diced fruit (such as orange sections),
    or pineapple chunks
3 ripe bananas, peeled

Bring the water to a boil; remove from the heat and add the raisins to soak until they are plump. Drain.

In a food processor or blender, process the raisins with the remaining ingredients until blended. Serve immediately.

---

1 SERVING = ¹⁄₄ CUP/60 mL = 1 FRUIT

PER SERVING:	total fat-0 g	sodium-1 mg	iron-0.4 mg
calories-74	(saturated fat-0 g)	potassium-284 mg	calcium-15 mg
protein-1 g	fiber-2.2 g	vitamin A-8 RE	phosphorus-20 mg
carbohydrates-19 g	cholesterol-0 mg	vitamin C-27 mg	

UMPERNICKEL BREAD

Makes 2 loaves or 24 slices (1 slice per serving)

1 tablespoon (15 mL) active dry yeast
3 tablespoons (45 mL) blackstrap molasses
2½ cups (625 mL) lukewarm water
2 cups (500 mL) whole-wheat flour
1 cup (250 mL) dark rye four

½ cup (125 mL) buckwheat flour
¼ cup (60 mL) cornmeal
2 tablespoons (30 mL) soy flour
1 teaspoon (5 mL) salt
2 cups (500 mL) whole-wheat flour
Oil as needed
Cornmeal for sprinkling

In a large mixing bowl, make a sponge by combining the yeast, molasses, water, and 2 cups of the whole-wheat flour. Whisk together until smooth; then set in a warm place for 10 minutes, until the mixture begins to bubble. Add the rye and buckwheat flours, cornmeal, soy flour and salt and stir to blend. Begin to add the final 2 cups of the wheat flour, ½ cup (125 mL) at a time.

When the dough is too stiff to keep stirring, turn it out onto a lightly floured surface, scraping the sides of the bowl clean. Knead for 10 minutes, adding enough flour to keep the dough from sticking to your hands.

Lightly oil the mixing bowl and return the kneaded dough to the bowl. Turn the dough over once to coat the top in oil. Set the dough aside to rise until doubled.

When the dough has risen, punch down and turn out onto work surface. Divide the dough in half. Form into oval loaves and place on a baking sheet that has been lightly sprinkled with the additional cornmeal. Let loaves rise again in warm place, covered with a damp tea towel or plastic wrap, until nearly double in bulk.

Preheat the oven to 350°F. When loaves have risen, bake for 45 minutes or until crust is browned and loaves sound hollow when tapped on the sides.

See glossary:

Blackstrap molasses
Buckwheat flour
Rye Flour, dark
Soy flour

1 SERVING = 1 SLICE = 1 GRAIN			
PER SLICE	total fat-1 g	sodium-92 mg	iron-1.5 mg
calories-103	(saturated fat-0 g)	potassium-186 mg	calcium-31 mg
protein-4 g	fiber-3.6 g	vitamin A-1 RE	phosphorus-97 mg
carbohydrates-22 g	cholesterol-0 mg	vitamin C- 0 mg	

SESAME RYE THINS

Makes 32 crackers (3 crackers per serving)

½ cup (125 mL) whole-wheat flour
½ cup (125 mL) rye flour
¼ cup (60 mL) oat bran
2 tablespoons (30 mL) sesame seeds
¼ teaspoon (1.2 mL) salt
2 tablespoons (30 mL) canola oil
1 tablespoon (15 mL) agave syrup or barley malt
¼ cup (60 mL) yogurt, soy or nonfat plain

Combine all the ingredients in a mixing bowl. Mix to form a smooth dough. Add more flour if the dough is sticky or more water if it is too dry.

Preheat the oven to 375°F. Press dough onto a baking sheet with your hands or roll it out with a floured rolling pin. With a sharp knife, cut the dough into 32 squares.

Bake for 10 to 15 minutes or until golden, checking during the last few minutes to be sure the crackers don't burn.

See glossary:

Agave syrup
Barley malt
Canola oil
Oat bran
Rye flour

1 SERVING = 3 CRACKERS = 1 GRAIN

PER CRACKER	total fat-1 g	sodium-17 mg	iron-0.2 mg
calories-26	(saturated fat-0 g)	potassium-21 mg	calcium-7 mg
protein-1 g	fiber-0.6 g	vitamin A-0 RE	phosphorus-16 mg
carbohydrates-3 g	cholesterol-0 mg	vitamin C-0 mg	

HERBED MUFFINS

Makes 12 muffins (1 muffin per serving)

These muffins taste like Thanksgiving stuffing.

1 medium onion, chopped

1 tablespoon (15 mL) tamari

2 tablespoons (30 mL) canola oil

1 tablespoon (15 mL) agave syrup
   or barley malt

¾ cup (185 mL) cooked couscous

1 cup (250 mL) soymilk or
   nonfat milk

1 cup (250 mL) barley flour

1 cup (250 mL) whole-wheat flour

1½ teaspoons (7.5 mL)
   baking soda

1½ teaspoons (7.5 mL)
   baking powder

½ teaspoon (2.5 mL) salt

1 teaspoon (5 mL) crushed
   dried rosemary

½ teaspoon (2.5 mL) dried thyme

1 teaspoon (5 mL) crushed
   dried sage

In a small skillet over medium heat, brown the onion with a few teaspoons of water and the tamari.

Preheat the oven to 350°F.

In a mixing bowl, combine the oil, syrup or malt, couscous, and soymilk or milk. Add the browned onion. Add the flours, baking soda, baking powder, salt, and herbs and stir until mixed. Spoon batter into a lightly oiled muffin pan. Bake for 20 minutes or until lightly browned and a toothpick inserted in the middle of the muffin comes out clean.

Remove from oven and cool completely before removing from the pan.

See glossary:

Agave syrup
Barley flour
Barley malt
Canola oil
Couscous
Soymilk
Tamari

1 SERVING = 1 MUFFIN = 1½ GRAINS

PER MUFFIN	total fat-3g	sodium-379 mg	iron-0.8 mg
calories-118	(saturated fat-0 g)	potassium-120 mg	calcium-52 mg
protein-4 g	fiber-3.5 g	vitamin A-1 RE	phosphorus-123 mg
carbohydrates-20 g	cholesterol-0 mg	vitamin C-1 mg	

APPLESAUCE-RAISIN MUFFINS

Makes 12 muffins (1 muffin per serving)

1 cup (250 mL) unsweetened applesauce

½ cup (125 mL) orange juice

2 tablespoons (30 mL) canola oil

1 tablespoon (15 mL) blackstrap molasses

2 tablespoons (30 mL) yogurt, soy or nonfat plain

1 cup (250 mL) whole-wheat flour

½ cup (125 mL) barley flour

½ cup (125 mL) rice flour

1½ teaspoons (7.5 mL) baking soda

½ teaspoon (2.5 mL) cinnamon

½ teaspoon (2.5 mL) salt

½ cup (125 mL) raisins

½ cup (125 mL) chopped walnuts

Preheat the oven to 350°F.

Combine the applesauce, orange juice, oil, molasses, and yogurt in a medium mixing bowl. Sift in the flours, baking soda, cinnamon, and salt. Mix just until moistened. Fold in the raisins and walnuts. Spoon into a lightly oiled muffin pan. Bake for 20 minutes or until lightly browned and a toothpick inserted in the middle of the muffin comes out clean. Let cool before removing from the pan.

See glossary:

Barley flour
Blackstrap molasses
Canola oil
Rice flour
Soy yogurt

1 SERVING = 1 MUFFIN = 1 GRAIN + ½ FRUIT + ½ NUT/SEED			
PER MUFFIN	total fat-6 g	sodium-25 mg	iron-1.2 mg
calories-163	(saturated fat-1 g)	potassium-223 mg	calcium-28 mg
protein-3 g	fiber-3.3 g	vitamin A-3 RE	phosphorus-86 mg
carbohydrates-27 g	cholesterol-0 mg	vitamin C-6 mg	

RISH-STYLE SCONES

Makes 12 scones (1 scone per serving)

Scones are the Irish version of American biscuits, only slightly sweeter.

¾ cup (185 mL) rice flour
¾ cup (185 mL) barley flour
½ cup (125 mL) whole-wheat flour
2 tablespoons (30 mL) ground flaxseed*
2 teaspoons (10 mL) baking powder
½ teaspoon (2.5 mL) salt
1½ tablespoons (22 mL) raw sugar
3 tablespoons (45 mL) canola oil
½ cup (125 mL) yogurt, soy or nonfat plain
½ cup (125 mL) raisins (optional)

In a medium mixing bowl, combine the flours, flaxseed, baking powder, salt, and sugar. Add the oil, yogurt, and raisins, if using. Mix until just moistened. Do not overmix.

Preheat the oven to 375°F.

On a lightly floured surface, pat the dough into a ½-inch-thick square. With a knife, cut the dough into triangles. Place the triangles on a baking sheet. Bake for 10 to 12 minutes, or until scones are golden brown.

*To grind flaxseed, place in an electric mill, such as the type used to grind coffee beans, and pulse until finely ground, or crush using a heavy mortar and pestle.

See glossary:

Barley flour
Canola oil
Flaxseed
Raw sugar
Rice flour
Soy yogurt

1 SERVING = 1 SCONE = 1 GRAIN + ½ NUT/SEED			
PER SCONE	total fat-5 g	sodium-153 mg	iron-0.8 mg
calories-127	(saturated fat-0 g)	potassium-89 mg	calcium-67 mg
protein-3 g	fiber-2.7 g	vitamin A-0 RE	phosphorus-146 mg
carbohydrates-19	cholesterol-0 mg	vitamin C-0 mg	

R ED CABBAGE SLAW

Serves 6 (²/₃ cup/165 mL per serving)

Our favorite addition to coleslaw is toasted sunflower seeds.
The crunch and flavor can't be beat.

½ cup (125 mL) chopped green onions
¼ cup (60 mL) minced fresh dill weed
⅓ cup (85 mL) toasted sunflower seeds
1 cup (250 mL) grated carrot
4 cups (1 L) grated red cabbage*
¼ cup (60 mL) lemon juice
⅓ cup (85 mL) Nayonaise, Veganaise, or other
    mayonnaise-like spread
Pinch of salt

To toast sunflower seeds, place in a heavy-bottomed skillet over high heat and stir until lightly browned, or roast the seeds on a baking sheet in a 400° F. oven or in a toaster oven for about 10 minutes, stirring several times. Take care that the seeds do not burn.

Combine the toasted sunflower seeds with all the other ingredients in a medium serving bowl.

*For more crunch in your slaw, chop the cabbage into thin strips. For a finer slaw, grate the cabbage on the coarse side of a grater.

1 SERVING = ²/₃ CUP/165 mL = 1 VEGETABLE + ½ NUT/SEED

PER SERVING	total fat-7 g	sodium-109 mg	iron-1 mg
calories-100	(saturated fat-0 g)	potassium-244 mg	calcium-44 mg
protein-3 g	fiber-2.6 g	vitamin A-521 RE	phosphorus-87 mg
carbohydrates-8 g	cholesterol-0 mg	vitamin C-35 mg	

GREEN SALAD WITH VINAIGRETTE

Serves 4 (1¹/₄ cups/310 mL per serving)

6 cups (1.5 L) mixed fresh greens
1 tablespoon (15 mL) flax oil
1 tablespoon (15 mL) extra-virgin olive oil
2 tablespoons (30 mL) balsamic vinegar
1 teaspoon (5 mL) tamari or miso
1 handful fresh herbs, roughly chopped
2 cloves garlic

Place the greens in a large salad bowl. Set aside.

In a food processor or blender, process the oils, vinegar, tamari or miso, herbs, and garlic until smooth. Pour over the salad and toss. Serve immediately.

See glossary:

Balsamic vinegar
Extra-virgin olive oil
Flax oil
Miso
Tamari

1 SERVING = 1¹/₄ CUPS/310 ML = 1 VEGETABLE + ¹/₂ NUT/SEED			
PER SERVING	total fat-7 g	sodium-120 mg	iron-1.8 mg
calories-78	(saturated fat-1 g)	potassium-344 mg	calcium-68 mg
protein-2 g	fiber-1.9 g	vitamin A-353 RE	phosphorus-33 mg
carbohydrates-3 g	cholesterol-0 mg	vitamin C- 19 mg	

Rich source of omega-3 fatty acids (providing at least 1 g per serving)

PICKLED CUCUMBERS
Serves 4 (½ cup/125 mL per serving)

2 cucumbers, sliced ¼ inch thick
¼ teaspoon (1.2 mL) salt
1 tablespoon (15 mL) flax oil
1½ tablespoons (22 mL) rice vinegar
     or apple cider vinegar
1 tablespoon (15 mL) water

Place the sliced cucumbers in a clean, dry 1-quart jar or bowl. Sprinkle with the salt. Pour the oil, vinegar, and water over the cucumbers. Refrigerate for at least an hour before serving.

See glossary:

Flax oil
Rice vinegar

1 SERVING = ½ CUP/125 mL = ½ VEGETABLE + ⅓ NUT/SEED

PER SERVING	total fat-4 g	sodium-136 mg	iron-0.4 mg
calories-50	(saturated fat-0 g)	potassium-222 mg	calcium-21 mg
protein-1 g	fiber-1.2 g	vitamin A-32 RE	phosphorus-31 mg
carbohydrates-4 g	cholesterol-0 mg	vitamin C-8 mg	

Rich source of omega-3 fatty acids (providing at least 1 g per serving)

FRESH SPINACH SALAD

Serves 5 (1½ cups (375/mL per serving)

⅓ cup (85 mL) raw almonds
5 cups (1.25 L) packed fresh spinach leaves, cleaned and
      torn into bite-sized pieces
2 carrots, grated
2 cloves garlic, minced
¼ cup (60 mL) lemon juice
1 teaspoon (5 mL) tamari
1 tablespoon (15 mL) toasted sesame oil
1 teaspoon (5 mL) extra-virgin olive oil

In a small dry skillet over high heat, toast the almonds, stirring, taking care not to burn. Remove the almonds from the skillet and set aside to cool.

Mix the spinach, grated carrots, and almonds together in a salad bowl. Set aside.

Shake the garlic, lemon juice, tamari, and oils together in a small jar. Pour the dressing over the salad. Toss well and serve immediately.

See glossary:

Extra-virgin olive oil
Tamari
Toasted sesame oil

1 SERVING = 1½ CUPS/375 mL = 1 VEGETABLE + 1 NUT/SEED			
PER SERVING	total fat-9 g	sodium-247 mg	iron-2.1 mg
calories-118	(saturated fat-1 g)	potassium-499 mg	calcium-90 mg
protein-4 g	fiber-3.5 g	vitamin A-1202 RE	phosphorus-95 mg
carbohydrates-8 g	cholesterol-0 mg	vitamin C-24 mg	

![S]WEET POTATO SALAD

Serves 6 (³/4 cup/185 mL per serving)

4 cups (1 L) peeled, cubed sweet potatoes
¼ cup (60 mL) chopped pecans
½ cup (125 mL) chopped green onion
2 tablespoons (30 mL) chopped cilantro
2 tablespoons (30 mL) light miso
¼ cup (60 mL) fresh lime juice

In a medium saucepan, steam the sweet potato cubes about 10 to 12 minutes or until tender but still firm enough to hold their shape. Drain and cool.

Combine the potatoes, pecans, green onion, and cilantro in a salad bowl.

In a cup or small bowl, mash the miso and lime juice together with a fork until creamy. Pour the miso mixture over the potato mixture. Mix gently but thoroughly.

See glossary:

Cilantro
Miso

1 SERVING = ³/4 CUP/185 mL = 1 GRAIN/STARCHY VEG + ½ NUT/SEED			
PER SERVING	total fat-4 g	sodium-175 mg	iron-0.7 mg
calories-152	(saturated fat-0 g)	potassium-389 mg	calcium-36 mg
protein-3 g	fiber-3.9 g	vitamin A-1994 RE	phosphorus-78 mg
carbohydrates-27 g	cholesterol-0 mg	vitamin C-28 mg	

NAVY BEAN MUSHROOM SOUP

Serves 5 (1¼ cups/310 mL per serving)

> *Use different kinds of mushrooms to vary this easy, creamy soup.*
> *Dry mushrooms that have been soaked in water or stock can*
> *be used to replace all or part of the fresh mushrooms.*

2 cups (500 mL) sliced mushrooms

2 medium onions, chopped

3 cloves garlic, minced

1 carrot, diced

2 teaspoons (10 mL) extra-virgin
   olive oil

2½ cups (625 mL) cooked,
   drained navy beans

3 cups (750 mL) bean cooking
   water or vegetable broth

¼ teaspoon (1.2 mL) dried thyme

¼ teaspoon (1.2 mL) dried savory

¼ teaspoon (1.2 mL) dried
   marjoram

½ teaspoon (2.5 mL) salt

Black pepper

In a medium skillet, sauté the mushrooms, onion, garlic, and carrots in the oil over medium heat for about 10 minutes, or until soft.

In a food processor or blender, process the beans with the stock or broth. (If you use a blender, do this in several batches.) Pour the purée into a soup pot and bring to a boil. Add the vegetables, thyme, savory, marjoram, salt, and pepper. Reduce the heat to a simmer and cook, covered, 5 minutes or until heated through.

Cooking Tip:	See glossary:
Buy legumes such as beans, lentils, garbanzo beans, and split peas when you know that you'll be needing them soon—very old beans take much longer to cook than fresh ones. Be sure to use up what you already have in the pantry before restocking.	Extra-virgin olive oil Marjoram Savory

1 SERVING = 1¼ CUPS/310 mL = 1¼ LEGUMES + 1 VEGETABLE

PER SERVING			
calories-179	total fat-3 g	sodium-222 mg	iron-2.8 mg
protein-9 g	(saturated fat-0 g)	potassium-567 mg	calcium-82 mg
carbohydrates-31 g	fiber-6.5 g	vitamin A-405 RE	phosphorus-197 mg
	cholesterol-0 mg	vitamin C-7 mg	

TRIPLE BEAN SOUP

Serves 6 (1¼ cups/310 mL per serving)

Fresh parsley and basil give this soup its special flavor.

2 teaspoons (10 mL) extra-virgin olive oil

1 cup (250 mL) chopped onion

1 green bell pepper, seeded, chopped

1 cup (250 mL) chopped celery

1 small jalapeño pepper, seeded, chopped (optional)*

3 cups (750 mL) stock or water

1 cup (250 mL) tomato purée

1 cup (250 mL) cooked, drained pinto beans

1 cup (250 mL) cooked, drained white beans

1 cup (250 mL) cooked, drained lima beans

2 tablespoons (30 mL) minced fresh basil

⅓ cup (85 mL) minced fresh parsley

2 teaspoons (10 mL) minced fresh cilantro

½ teaspoon (2.5 mL) salt (optional)

Black pepper

½ cup (125 mL) sunflower seeds

In a soup pot, heat the oil. Sauté the onion, bell pepper, celery, and jalapeño, if using, over medium heat about 10 minutes or until soft, stirring frequently. Add the stock or broth, tomatoes, beans, basil, parsley, cilantro, salt, if using, and black pepper. Bring to a boil, reduce the heat, and simmer for 10 to 15 minutes or until heated through.

While the soup cooks, toast the sunflower seeds in a small, dry skillet over high heat, stirring often, taking care not to burn. Coarsely grind the toasted seeds in a food processor or blender.

Ladle the soup into serving bowls. Garnish with the ground seeds.

*Be sure to wear gloves when handling hot peppers to prevent skin irritation.

See glossary:

Cilantro
Extra-virgin olive oil
Jalapeño pepper

1 SERVING = 1¼ CUPS/310 mL = 1½ LEGUMES + ½ NUT/SEED + ½ VEG

PER SERVING	total fat-8 g	sodium-265 mg	iron-3.8 mg
calories-239	(saturated fat-1 g)	potassium-778 mg	calcium-93 mg
protein-12 g	fiber-9.8 g	vitamin A-49 RE	phosphorus-254 mg
carbohydrates-32 g	cholesterol-0 mg	vitamin C-29 mg	

BLACK-EYED PEAS AND GREENS SOUP

Serves 6 (1¼ cups/310 mL per serving)

1 tablespoon (15 mL) extra-virgin olive oil
2 tablespoons (30 mL) chopped garlic
1 large green bell pepper, seeded, chopped
1 jalapeño pepper, seeded, minced*
4 cups (1 L) chopped fresh greens, such as collards, kale,
　　and/or mustard greens
5 cups (1.25 L) stock or water
3 cups (750 mL) cooked, drained black-eyed peas
¼ cup (60 mL) dark miso**
1 cup (250 mL) warm water

In a soup pot, heat the olive oil. Sauté the garlic, bell pepper, and jalapeño pepper over medium heat about 5 minutes or until tender, stirring occasionally. Add the greens and stock or water. Bring to a boil. Lower the heat and simmer for 15 minutes. Add the black-eyed peas and return to a boil. Lower the heat to a simmer.

While soup simmers, dissolve the miso in the cup of warm water. Turn off the heat under the soup and add the miso mixture. Stir to blend.

*Be sure to wear gloves when handling hot peppers to prevent skin irritation.

**Be sure to add miso when the soup is below the boiling point, so the enzymes in the miso will not be destroyed.

See glossary:

Extra-virgin olive oil
Jalapeño pepper
Kale
Miso
Mustard greens

1 SERVING = 1¼ CUPS/310 mL = 1¼ LEGUMES + 1 VEGETABLE			
PER SERVING	total fat-4 g	sodium-441 mg	iron-3.4 mg
calories-174	(saturated fat-1 g)	potassium-510 mg	calcium-103 mg
protein-10 g	fiber-7.4 g	vitamin A-417 RE	phosphorus-188 mg
carbohydrates-28 g	cholesterol-0 mg	vitamin C-68 mg	

STUFFED ZUCCHINI

Serves 6 (½ zucchini plus stuffing per serving)

3 zucchini, about 8 to10 inches long
1 cup (250 mL) raw cashew pieces
1 teaspoon (5 mL) extra-virgin
 olive oil
2 tablespoons (30 mL) minced
 garlic
1½ cups (375 mL) green peas
⅓ cup (85 mL) chopped fresh
 parsley

3 cups (750 mL) cooked millet,
 barley, brown rice, or kasha
1 medium onion, chopped
1 (28-ounce/794 mL) can crushed
 tomatoes or 3½ cups (875 mL)
 crushed fresh tomatoes
2 tablespoons (30 mL) grated
 gingerroot

Cut the zucchini in half lengthwise. Scoop out the seeds, leaving ¼ to ½ inch of the squash intact with the skin. Steam the squash in a little water in a large covered saucepan for 8 to 10 minutes.

While the zucchini steams, toast the cashews in a small, dry skillet over high heat, stirring until lightly browned and taking care not to burn.

In the same skillet, heat the oil. Sauté the garlic in the oil over medium-low heat for 1 minute. Add the peas and stir for several minutes. Add the parsley and cooked grain, and stir together over low heat until heated through.

To prepare the sauce, steam the onion in 2 tablespoons (30 mL) water in a medium saucepan over medium-high heat. Stir to keep the onion from sticking. Add the tomatoes and gingerroot, and heat through.

Preheat the oven to 400°F. To assemble, place the squash cut side up in a rectangular baking dish. Spoon the grain mixture into the squash, and press to fill all six pieces evenly. Pour the tomato sauce over the zucchini. Bake for 15 minutes, then lower the heat to 350° F, and bake for an additional 20 minutes.

See glossary:

Barley
Brown rice
Extra-virgin olive oil
Kasha
Millet

1 SERVING = 1 LEGUME + 1 NUT/SEED + 1½ GRAINS + 1 VEGETABLE

PER SERVING	total fat-14 g	sodium-31 mg	iron-4.2 mg
calories-377	(saturated fat-3 g)	potassium-892 mg	calcium-80 mg
protein-12 g	fiber-7.4 g	vitamin A-141 RE	phosphorus-355 mg
carbohydrates-54 g	cholesterol-0 mg	vitamin C-45 mg	

OVEN BAKED VEGGIES WITH GOLDEN SAUCE

Serves 4 (1½ cups/375 mL per serving)

1 teaspoon (5 mL) extra-virgin olive oil
1 large red bell pepper, seeded
2 stalks broccoli
1 large onion
½ pound (227 g) mushrooms
1 tablespoon (15 mL) tamari
1 cup (250 mL) buckwheat groats
2½ cups (625 mL) water

Preheat the oven to 450°F. Spread the oil over a large baking sheet. Chop the vegetables into large bite-sized pieces, and spread the vegetables evenly over the baking sheet; sprinkle with tamari. Bake for 15 minutes. Turn the vegetables over with a spatula and bake 10 more minutes, or until lightly browned.

While the vegetables roast, make kasha by toasting the buckwheat groats in a dry skillet over high heat until golden, stirring frequently and taking care not to burn. Add the water to the skillet, cover, and simmer for 20 minutes, or until the water is absorbed and the kasha is tender. Remove from the heat and leave covered for a few more minutes.

GOLDEN SAUCE

¾ cup (185 mL) nutritional yeast flakes

1 teaspoon (5 mL) garlic powder

1 teaspoon (5 mL) ground cumin

½ teaspoon (2.5 mL) turmeric

¼ cup (60 mL) arrowroot

2 tablespoons (30 mL) spicy mustard

2 cups (500 mL) soymilk or nonfat milk

Salt and black pepper

While the kasha cooks, make the sauce by combining the yeast flakes, garlic powder, cumin, turmeric, and arrowroot in a medium saucepan. Whisk in the mustard and soymilk, and cook over medium heat, stirring, until the sauce thickens. To serve, top the kasha with the vegetables and sauce.

See glossary:

Arrowroot

Extra-virgin olive oil

Kasha

Nutritional yeast flakes

Soymilk

Tamari

Turmeric

1 SERVING = 1½ CUPS/375 mL = 1¼ LEGUMES + 1 GRAIN + 2 VEGETABLES

PER SERVING	total fat-5 g	sodium-296 mg	iron-3 mg
calories-268	(saturated fat-1 g)	potassium-991 mg	calcium-54 mg
protein-20 g	fiber-6.4 g	vitamin A-141 RE	phosphorus-428 mg
carbohydrates-45 g	cholesterol-0 mg	vitamin C-65 mg	

ARUGULA AND GARBANZO BEAN SALAD

Serves 6 (1 cup/250 mL per serving)

1 cup (250 mL) barley
2½ cups (625 mL) water
2 cups (500 mL) cooked, drained
  garbanzo beans
¾ cup (185 mL) chopped celery
¾ cup (185 mL) chopped, seeded
  red bell pepper
½ cup (125 mL) chopped fresh
  parsley
3 cups (750 mL) chopped arugula,
  kale, mustard, or other dark
  leafy greens

DRESSING
2 cloves garlic, minced
1 teaspoon (5 mL) toasted
  sesame oil
1 tablespoon (15 mL) extra-virgin
  olive oil or hempseed oil
1 tablespoon (15 mL) rice vinegar
1 tablespoon (15 mL) balsamic
  vinegar
Salt and black pepper

Bring the barley and water to a boil in a covered medium saucepan. Reduce the heat and let simmer for 20 to 25 minutes, or until the water is absorbed and the barley is tender. Remove from the heat and let sit covered until cool.

In large bowl, mix together the garbanzo beans, celery, red bell pepper, parsley, and arugula or other greens. Add the cooled barley and mix together.

In a small jar, shake together all the dressing ingredients. Pour the dressing over the salad, and mix well.

See glossary:

Arugula
Balsamic vinegar
Barley
Extra-virgin olive oil
Garbanzo beans
Hempseed oil
Kale
Mustard greens
Rice vinegar
Toasted sesame oil

1 SERVING = 1 CUP/250 mL = 1 GRAIN + ¾ LEGUME + ½ NUT/SEED + 1 VEG

PER SERVING			
calories-242	total fat-5 g	sodium-28 mg	iron-3.5 mg
protein-8 g	(saturated fat-1 g)	potassium-421 mg	calcium-64 mg
carbohydrates-44 g	fiber-8 g	vitamin A-153 RE	phosphorus-158 mg
	cholesterol-0 mg	vitamin C-34 mg	

B ARLEY AND LENTIL STEW

Serves 6 (1½ cups/375 mL per serving)

¾ cup (185 mL) barley
¾ cup (185 mL) lentils
6 cups (1.5 L) water
1 large bay leaf
3 cups (750 mL) peeled, cubed sweet potatoes
3 cups (750 mL) chopped kale
1 head of garlic, cloves peeled and minced
½ teaspoon (2.5 mL) dried rosemary
2 tablespoons (30 mL) dark miso
¼ cup (60 mL) water
3 tablespoons (45 mL) toasted sesame seeds

In a large covered pot, bring the barley and lentils to a boil in the 6 cups (1.5 L) of water. Reduce the heat and simmer for 40 minutes, or until the water is absorbed and the barley and lentils are tender. Add the sweet potatoes, kale, garlic, and rosemary. Cook for 15 more minutes, or until the potatoes are soft, adding more water if necessary.

Remove from the heat. Stir the miso into the ¼ cup (60 mL) water, and add to the stew. Mix well, cover the pot, and let set for several minutes.

To toast the sesame seeds, cook in a small, hot, dry skillet over high heat, stirring, until golden, taking care not to burn. Just before serving, sprinkle the stew with the toasted sesame seeds.

See glossary:

Barley
Kale
Miso

---

1 SERVING = 1½ CUPS/375 mL = 2 GRAINS/STARCHY VEG + 1 VEG + 1 LEGUME

PER SERVING	total fat-4 g	sodium-242 mg	iron-4.6 mg
calories-312	(saturated fat-1 g)	potassium-630 mg	calcium-134 mg
protein-10 g	fiber-10.8 g	vitamin A-2168 RE	phosphorus-212 mg
carbohydrates-62 g	cholesterol-0 mg	vitamin C-60 mg	

LENTIL PIE

Serves 8 (1½ cups/375 mL per serving)

3 cups (750 mL) cooked, cubed white potato

1 tablespoon plus 1 teaspoon (20 mL) extra-virgin olive oil

½ cup (125 mL) soymilk or nonfat milk

Black pepper

2 tablespoons (30 mL) white miso

4 cups (1 L) cooked, cubed sweet potato

1 medium onion, chopped

1 green bell pepper, seeded, chopped

2 tablespoons (30 mL) minced garlic or 1 teaspoon (5 mL) garlic powder

1 large carrot, chopped

2 cups (500 mL) tomato purée

3 cups (750 mL) cooked, drained, lentils

¼ teaspoon (1.2 mL) dried thyme

½ teaspoon (2.5 mL) dried marjoram

½ teaspoon (2.5 mL) salt (optional)

Paprika for garnish

In a small saucepan, mash the white potatoes with the 1 tablespoon (15 mL) olive oil, ¼ cup (60 mL) of the soymilk, black pepper, and 1 tablespoon (15 mL) of the miso. Set aside.

In a separate saucepan, mash the sweet potatoes with the remaining ¼ cup (60 mL) soymilk, black pepper, and the remaining 1 tablespoon (15 mL) miso. Set aside.

In a large pot, heat the 1 teaspoon (5 mL) olive oil over medium heat. Sauté the onion, green bell pepper, garlic, and carrot in the oil for 5 minutes, stirring occasionally. Add the tomato purée, lentils, thyme, marjoram, and salt, if using, and bring to a boil. Remove the mixture from the heat, and pour into a 9 x 13-inch baking dish.

Preheat the oven to 350°F. With your hands or a large spoon, spread half the white potato over one-quarter of the pie. Next to that, put half the sweet potato, followed by the rest of the white potato and the rest of the sweet potato. Sprinkle the pie with paprika, and bake for 45 minutes. Let cool for 10 minutes before serving.

See glossary:

Extra-virgin olive oil

Miso

Soymilk

1 SERVING = 1 LEGUME + 1 GRAIN/STARCHY VEG + 1 VEGETABLE + ¼ NUT/SEED

PER SERVING	total fat-3 g	sodium-124 mg	iron-3.4 mg
calories-235	(saturated fat-0 g)	potassium-852 mg	calcium-52 mg
protein-10 g	fiber-9.9 g	vitamin A-1229 RE	phosphorus-215 mg
carbohydrates-43 g	cholesterol-0 mg	vitamin C-38 mg	

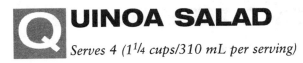UINOA SALAD

Serves 4 (1¼ cups/310 mL per serving)

1 cup (250 mL) quinoa
1½ cups (375 mL) water
1 cup (250 mL) cooked, drained kidney beans
1 fresh tomato, chopped
1 cucumber, seeded, chopped
1 large carrot, diced
½ cup (125 mL) chopped green onion
½ cup (125 mL) chopped fresh parsley
1 tablespoon (15 mL) minced fresh basil
    or 1 teaspoon (5 mL) dried basil
2 cloves garlic, minced
¼ cup (60 mL) rice vinegar
1 tablespoon (15 mL) unsweetened apple juice
1 tablespoon (15 mL) toasted sesame oil
1 tablespoon (15 mL) tamari or Bragg Liquid Aminos

Bring the quinoa and water to a boil in a medium saucepan. Reduce the heat to a simmer, and cook for 10 to 15 minutes or until the quinoa is tender and the water is absorbed. Turn the quinoa out onto a baking sheet and let cool.

In a serving bowl, combine the beans, tomato, cucumber, carrot, green onion, parsley, and basil. Add the garlic, vinegar, apple juice, sesame oil, and tamari or liquid aminos; mix well. Add the cooled quinoa and stir to combine with the vegetables and dressing.

See glossary:

Bragg Liquid Aminos
Quinoa
Rice vinegar
Toasted sesame oil
Tamari

---

1 SERVING = 1¼ CUPS/310 mL = 1 GRAIN + 1 LEGUME + 1 VEG + ½ NUT/SEED

PER SERVING	total fat-6 g	sodium-278 mg	iron-6.5 mg
calories-282	(saturated fat-1 g)	potassium-830 mg	calcium-76 mg
protein-11 g	fiber-7.4 g	vitamin A-584 RE	phosphorus-283 mg
carbohydrates-48 g	cholesterol-0 mg	vitamin C-24 mg	

OLENTA-TEMPEH BAKE

Serves 8 (1¼ cups/310 mL per serving)

1 cup (250 mL) coarsely ground
  cornmeal
3⅓ cups (835 mL) water
¼ teaspoon (1.2 mL) salt (optional)
1 tablespoon (15 mL) extra-virgin
  olive oil, divided
1 pound (454 g) tempeh, cut into
  ½-inch cubes
2 teaspoons (10 mL) tamari
1 large green bell pepper, seeded,
  chopped

1 large onion, chopped
1 tablespoon (15 mL) chopped
  garlic
1 (28-ounce/794 mL) can crushed
  tomatoes or 3½ cups (875 mL)
  crushed fresh tomatoes
1 (6-ounce/168 mL) can tomato
  paste
½ cup (125 mL) lemon juice
2 tablespoons (30 mL) dried basil
½ teaspoon (2.5 mL) salt (optional)

In a medium saucepan, add the cornmeal and salt, if using, to the water and bring to a boil. Reduce the heat to medium-low and cook, stirring often to prevent sticking, about 15 minutes or until polenta is thick.

Lightly oil a 9 x 13-inch baking dish with 1 teaspoon (5 mL) of the oil. Pour the polenta into the dish. Set aside to cool.

Preheat the oven to 350°F. Lightly oil a baking sheet with 1 teaspoon (5 mL) of the oil. Place the tempeh on the baking sheet and sprinkle with the tamari. Bake for 15 minutes. Flip the tempeh over and bake another 15 minutes.

Heat the remaining 1 teaspoon (5 mL) oil in a large saucepan. Sauté the bell pepper, onion, and garlic over medium heat, about 5 minutes or until soft. Add the tomatoes, tomato paste, lemon juice, basil, and salt, if using. Simmer sauce for 5 to 10 minutes.

---

1 SERVING = 1½ CUPS/375 mL = 1 LEGUME + 1 GRAIN + 1 VEGETABLE

PER SERVING	total fat-7 g	sodium-163 mg	iron-3 mg
calories-237	(saturated fat-1 g)	potassium-748 mg	calcium-96 mg
protein-14 g	fiber-7.1 g	vitamin A-131 RE	phosphorus-201 mg
carbohydrates-33 g	cholesterol-0 mg	vitamin C-37 mg	

When the polenta is cool and firm, slice it into bite-sized squares. With a spatula, loosen the squares from the baking dish. Place the tempeh cubes in and around the polenta squares. Pour the tomato sauce over the tempeh and polenta. Bake for 25 minutes. Let cool about 10 minutes before serving.

See glossary:

Extra-virgin olive oil
Polenta
Tamari
Tempeh

TOFU SALAD DELIGHT

Serves 5 (¹/₂ cup/125 mL per serving)

This salad got raves when it was served to guests who were not vegetarian or familiar with eating tofu. They had to get the recipe so they could enjoy it again.

1 pound (454 g) tofu, divided
1 tablespoon (15 mL) toasted sesame seeds
¹/₂ cup (125 mL) chopped green onions, tops and bottoms
¹/₄ cup (60 mL) fresh dill, minced
1 tablespoon (15 mL) tamari

1 tablespoon (15 mL) apple cider vinegar
¹/₂ tablespoon (7 mL) spicy mustard
3 tablespoons (45 mL) nayonaise (or other mayonnaise-like spread)
¹/₂ stalk celery, finely chopped

Crumble half of the tofu in a mixing bowl. Process the other half of the tofu in a food processor or blender until smooth. Add to the bowl with the remaining ingredients, and mix well. Serve with raw vegetables as dippers or spread on rice cakes, crackers, or corn chips.

1 SERVING = ¹/₂ CUP/125 mL = 1 LEGUME + ¹/₂ NUT/SEED			
PER SERVING	total fat-11 g	sodium-310 mg	iron-10.1 mg
calories-171	(saturated fat-1 g)	potassium-295 mg	calcium-216 mg
protein-15 g	fiber-2.8 g	vitamin A-21 RE	phosphorus-195 mg
carbohydrates-6 g	cholesterol-0 mg	vitamin C-3 mg	

VEGETABLE SKEWERS

Serves 6 (1 skewer per serving)

*Plan ahead so you can marinate the tofu either overnight or all day.
The skewers can be grilled over coals or baked in the oven.*

½ cup (125 mL) vegetable stock
1 head garlic, cloves peeled
1 tablespoon (15 mL) extra-virgin olive oil
1 tablespoon (15 mL) toasted sesame oil
1½ tablespoons (22 mL) balsamic vinegar
2 tablespoons (30 mL) tamari
1½ pounds (681 g) firm tofu, cut into ½-inch cubes
½ pound (227 g) mushrooms
1 green bell pepper, seeded, cut into wedges
1 red bell pepper, seeded, cut into wedges
3 medium zucchini, thickly sliced
2 medium onions, peeled, quartered

In a blender, combine the stock, garlic cloves, oils, vinegar, and tamari.
Place the marinade and tofu in a shallow dish. Cover and refrigerate for at
least 6 hours.

Preheat the oven to 350°F. To assemble, thread 6 skewers with the marinated tofu and vegetables, alternating colors and repeating until the skewers are filled. Place skewers on a baking sheet and baste with the remaining marinade. Bake for 20 minutes. Turn once and bake for another 15 minutes. If grilling, cook over a hot grill, turning once, until each side of the skewers is crispy and the squash and onions are tender.

See glossary:

Balsamic vinegar
Extra-virgin olive oil
Tamari
Toasted sesame oil
Tofu

1 SERVING = 1 SKEWER = 1⅓ LEGUMES + ½ NUT/SEED + 2 VEGETABLES

PER SERVING	total fat-15 g	sodium-356 mg	iron-13 mg
calories-257	(saturated fat-2 g)	potassium-673 mg	calcium-262 mg
protein-21 g	fiber-5 g	vitamin A-88 RE	phosphorus-305 mg
carbohydrates-16 g	cholesterol-0 mg	vitamin C-42 mg	

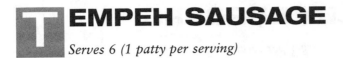

TEMPEH SAUSAGE

Serves 6 (1 patty per serving)

*Tempeh Sausages keep well refrigerated or frozen,
so make them ahead of time.*

½ pound (227 g) tempeh
¼ cup (60 mL) water (reserved from steaming the tempeh)
1 tablespoon (15 mL) extra-virgin olive oil
1 tablespoon (15 mL) dark miso
2 tablespoons (30 mL) rolled oats
¼ teaspoon (1.2 mL) garlic powder
¼ teaspoon (1.2 mL) dried thyme
½ teaspoon (2.5 mL) dried sage
2 tablespoons (30 mL) nutritional yeast flakes
Black pepper

Steam the tempeh over simmering water for 10 minutes. Remove from the pan and cool. (Keep ¼ cup/60 mL of the cooking water to add to the sausage later.)

When cool, grate the tempeh into a medium mixing bowl. Add the remaining ingredients, including the ¼ cup/60 mL of the reserved water from steaming, and mix well. Shape into 6 patties, pressing very firmly, and cook in a lightly oiled skillet over medium-high heat 5 to 6 minutes, turning once, or until lightly browned.

See glossary:

Extra-virgin olive oil
Miso
Nutritional yeast flakes
Oats, rolled
Tempeh

1 SERVING = 1 PATTY = 1 LEGUME

PER SERVING	total fat-6 g	sodium-108 mg	iron-1.1 mg
calories-115	(saturated fat-1 g)	potassium-203 mg	calcium-40 mg
protein-9 g	fiber-2.4 g	vitamin A-27 RE	phosphorus-119 mg
carbohydrates-9 g	cholesterol-0 mg	vitamin C-0 mg	

BARLEY BURGERS

Serves 6 (1 burger per serving)

½ cup (125 mL) barley
1½ cups (375 mL) water
½ cup (125 mL) walnuts
2 tablespoons (30 mL) ground
  flaxseed*
½ cup (125 mL) minced onion

1 small zucchini, grated
½ cup (125 mL) chopped fresh
  parsley
1 teaspoon (5 mL) dried basil
2 tablespoons (30 mL) tahini
1 tablespoon (15 mL) tamari

Bring the barley and water to a boil in a covered medium saucepan. Lower the heat and simmer for 25 minutes or until the barley is tender and the water is absorbed.

While the barley cooks, process the walnuts in a food processor or blender to make a coarse meal. Combine the walnut meal, flaxseed, onion, zucchini, parsley, basil, tahini, and tamari in a mixing bowl. Add the hot barley and stir to combine.

Preheat the oven to 400°F. Using a large spoon, drop the barley mixture onto a lightly oiled baking sheet. Shape the mixture to form patties. Bake for 25 to 30 minutes or until lightly browned, turning once.

*To grind flaxseed, place in an electric mill, such as the type used to grind coffee beans, and pulse until finely ground, or crush using a heavy mortar and pestle.

See glossary:

Barley
Flaxseed
Tahini
Tamari

Cooking Tip:

Rice is a familiar ingredient to us all but have you tried other grains? Whole grains combine well with beans. After they are cooked, they are good in soups, stews, hot cereal, salads, and added to bread dough or baked goods.

1 SERVING = 1 BURGER = 1 GRAIN + ¾ NUT/SEED

PER SERVING	total fat-9 g	sodium-152 mg	iron-1.5 mg
calories-151	(saturated fat-1 g)	potassium-194 mg	calcium-49 mg
protein-4 g	fiber-3.4 g	vitamin A-28 RE	phosphorus-109 mg
carbohydrates-17 g	cholesterol-0 mg	vitamin C-8 mg	

Rich source of omega-3 fatty acids (providing at least 1 g per serving)

BAKED SQUASH CASSEROLE

Serves 4 (³/4 cup/185 mL per serving)

Butternut, hubbard, acorn, or any other orange-fleshed squash makes this dish a sweet accompaniment to your main course.

3 cups (750 mL) peeled, cubed squash
¹/2 cup (125 mL) orange juice
¹/2 cup (125 mL) chopped dried apricots
3 tablespoons (45 mL) ground flaxseed*
¹/4 teaspoon (1.2 mL) salt (optional)

Steam the squash in a covered saucepan in ¹/4 inch of water for about 10 minutes, until tender. Drain the water and mash the squash lightly with a fork, leaving some chunks.

Preheat the oven to 350°F. Put the squash into a small baking dish, and add the remaining ingredients. Stir thoroughly, cover, and bake for 20 minutes.

*To grind flaxseed, place in an electric mill, such as the type used to grind coffee beans, and pulse until finely ground, or crush using a heavy mortar and pestle.

See glossary:

Flaxseed

---

1 SERVING = ³/4 CUP/185 mL = 1 GRAIN/STARCHY VEGETABLE + 1 FRUIT

PER SERVING	total fat-2 g	sodium-8 mg	iron-1.9 mg
calories-125	(saturated fat-0 g)	potassium-676 mg	calcium-84 mg
protein-3 g	fiber-6.6 g	vitamin A-1151 RE	phosphorus-84 mg
carbohydrates-28 g	cholesterol-0 mg	vitamin C-39 mg	

Rich source of omega-3 fatty acids (providing at least 1 g per serving)

GREEN BEANS WITH LEMON AND DILL

Serves 4 (³/4 cup/185 mL per serving)

4 cups (1 L) bite-sized pieces green beans
2 tablespoons (30 mL) water
3 tablespoons (45 mL) slivered almonds
Juice of one lemon
¼ cup (60 mL) minced fresh dill weed
    or 1 tablespoon (15 mL) dried dill weed
1 teaspoon (5 mL) light miso

In a medium saucepan over medium-high heat, steam the green beans in the 2 tablespoons (30 mL) water for 2 minutes. Lower the heat and add the almonds, lemon juice, and dill. Simmer for 1 more minute.

Turn off the heat and stir the miso into the liquid in the bottom of the pan. Cover and let sit for several minutes before serving.

See glossary:

Miso

1 SERVING = ³/4 CUP/185 mL = 1 VEGETABLE + ¹/2 NUT/SEED

PER SERVING	total fat-4 g	sodium-110 mg	iron-1.4 mg
calories-88	(saturated fat-0 g)	potassium-302 mg	calcium-60 mg
protein-4 g	fiber-4.8 g	vitamin A-74 mg	phosphorus-84 mg
carbohydrates-12g	cholesterol-0 mg	vitamin C-23 mg	

GINGERED GARBANZO BEANS

Serves 6 (1¼ cups/310 mL per serving)

For a hearty main dish, serve Gingered Garbanzo Beans over brown rice, millet, or quinoa.

1 teaspoon (5 mL) extra-virgin olive oil

1 medium onion, chopped

1 tablespoon (15 mL) minced garlic

1 head bok choy, chopped

1 (28-ounce/794 mL) can crushed tomatoes

    or 3½ cups (875 mL) crushed fresh tomatoes

2 tablespoons (30 mL) grated gingerroot

3 cups (750 mL) cooked, drained garbanzo beans

Salt (optional)

Black pepper

Heat the oil in a large skillet. Sauté the onion, garlic, and bok choy in the oil over medium heat 5 minutes or until soft.

Add the tomatoes, gingerroot, and garbanzo beans, and bring to a boil. Reduce the heat and simmer for a few minutes. Season with salt, if using, and black pepper.

Cooking Tip:	See glossary:
Adding bay leaves, garlic, and other herbs can enhance the flavor of cooked beans. Acidic foods such as tomatoes, lemon juice, vinegar, and wine can toughen the skin of cooking beans so add them after the beans are soft.	Bok choy Extra-virgin olive oil Garbanzo beans Gingerroot

1 SERVING = 1¼ CUPS/310 mL = 1 LEGUME + 2 VEGETABLES

PER SERVING	total fat-3 g	sodium-54 mg	iron-3.6 mg
calories-185	(saturated fat-0 g)	potassium-698 mg	calcium-129 mg
protein-10 g	fiber-7 g	vitamin A-222 RE	phosphorus-189 mg
carbohydrates-32 g	cholesterol-0 mg	vitamin C-44 mg	

SPICY CABBAGE

Serves 6 (½ cup/125 mL per serving)

1 tablespoon (15 mL) extra-virgin olive oil
½ teaspoon (2.5 mL) chili powder
2 teaspoons (10 mL) grated gingerroot
1 teaspoon (5 mL) crushed yellow mustard seed
½ teaspoon (2.5 mL) turmeric
1 large onion, chopped
3 cloves garlic, minced
1 tablespoon (15 mL) water
1 head green cabbage, cored, chopped
1 tablespoon (15 mL) barley malt
2 tablespoons (30 mL) apple cider vinegar
¼ cup (60 mL) chopped walnuts

Heat the oil in a large skillet over medium-high heat. Add the chili powder, gingerroot, mustard seed, and turmeric and cook, stirring constantly, about 1 minute or until aromatic, taking care not to burn.

Lower the heat to medium and add the onions, garlic, water, and cabbage. Cover and cook for 10 to 15 minutes, stirring occasionally. Add the barley malt, vinegar, and walnuts and stir. Cover and cook a minute or two until heated through.

See glossary:

Barley malt
Extra-virgin olive oil
Gingerroot
Turmeric

1 SERVING = ½ CUP/125 mL = 2 VEGETABLES + ½ NUT/SEED

PER SERVING			
calories-100	total fat-6 g	sodium-10 mg	iron-0.4 mg
protein-2 g	(saturated fat-1 g)	potassium-201 mg	calcium-44 mg
carbohydrates-11 g	fiber-3.8 g	vitamin A-14 RE	phosphorus-53 mg
	cholesterol-0 mg	vitamin C-23 mg	

MARINATED VEGETABLES

Serves 6 (²/₃ cup/165 mL per serving)

*These crisp vegetables are great to have on hand
as a quick snack or accompaniment to a meal.*

¹/₂ teaspoon (2.5 mL) dill seed or 1 bunch fresh dill weed

¹/₂ teaspoon (2.5 mL) mustard seed

1 cup (250 mL) thickly sliced carrots

1 cup (250 mL) roughly chopped cauliflower

1 cup (250 mL) cut-up green beans

1 cup (250 mL) sliced zucchini

3 cloves garlic, chopped

¹/₂ cup (125 mL) apple cider vinegar

³/₄ cup (185 mL) water

1 teaspoon (5 mL) salt

Put the dill seed or dill weed and mustard seed in a clean, dry 1-quart glass jar with a tight-fitting lid. Pack the vegetables and garlic into the jar. Set aside.

In a small saucepan, bring the vinegar, water, and salt to a boil. Remove from the heat and pour the mixture over the vegetables. Screw on the lid and set the jar aside to cool.

When cool, refrigerate the jar for several days to marinate the vegetables before serving.

1 SERVING = ²/₃ CUP/165 mL = 1 VEGETABLE

PER SERVING	total fat-0 g	sodium-367 mg	iron-0.6 mg
calories-25	(saturated fat-0 g)	potassium-213 mg	calcium-24 mg
protein-1 g	fiber-1.7 g	vitamin A-357 RE	phosphorus-33 mg
carbohydrates-6 g	cholesterol-0 mg	vitamin C- 15 mg	

OAT AND APPLE COOKIES

Makes 24 cookies (1 cookie per serving)

1 cup (250 mL) grated apple

1 tablespoon (15 mL) ground
flaxseed*

⅓ cup (85 mL) unsweetened
applesauce

½ cup (125 mL) chopped dried
apricots

2 tablespoons (30 mL) canola oil

¼ cup (60 mL) maple syrup

½ teaspoon (2.5 mL) vanilla
extract

½ cup (125 mL) walnuts

1 cup (250 mL) rolled oats

1 teaspoon (5 mL) baking powder

1 teaspoon (5 mL) cinnamon

¼ teaspoon (1.2 mL) salt
(optional)

Mix the apple, flaxseed, applesauce, apricots, oil, syrup, and vanilla together in a large bowl. In a food processor or blender, process the walnuts into a coarse meal, and add to the apple mixture.

In the same food processor or blender, process the oats to the texture of coarse flour. Add the baking powder, cinnamon, and salt, if using, and process briefly to blend. Mix the oat mixture in the bowl with the apple mixture.

Preheat the oven to 350°F. Drop dough by the teaspoonful onto a baking sheet. Bake for 15 minutes, or until golden brown on the bottom. Remove from the oven and let sit 1 to 2 minutes on the baking sheet to firm slightly. Remove the cookies to a wire rack, and cool completely.

*To grind flaxseed, place in an electric mill, such as the type used to grind coffee beans, and pulse until finely ground, or crush using a heavy mortar and pestle.

See glossary:

Canola oil
Flaxseed
Oats, rolled

1 SERVING = 1 COOKIE = ¾ GRAIN

PER SERVING	total fat-3 g	sodium-16 mg	iron-0.4 mg
calories-61	(saturated fat-0 g)	potassium-79 mg	calcium-23 mg
protein-1 g	fiber-1 g	vitamin A-21 RE	phosphorus-48 mg
carbohydrates-8 g	cholesterol-0 mg	vitamin C-1 mg	

APPLE CRISP

Serves 6 (²/₃ cup/165 mL per serving)

5 cups (1.25 mL) sliced apples
2 tablespoons (30 mL) lemon juice
½ teaspoon (2.5 mL) cinnamon
1½ tablespoons (22 mL) agave syrup or honey
1½ cups (375 mL) rolled oats
¼ cup (60 mL) chopped walnuts
¼ cup (60 mL) sunflower seeds
1 teaspoon (5 mL) vanilla extract
2 tablespoons (30 mL) water
1½ tablespoons (22 mL) agave syrup or maple syrup

Preheat the oven to 350°F.

Layer the apples in an 8 x 8-inch baking dish along with the lemon juice, cinnamon, and 1½ tablespoons (22 mL) of the agave syrup. Press down the top to flatten.

In a separate bowl, combine the oats, walnuts, sunflower seeds, vanilla, water, and 1½ tablespoons (22 mL) of the agave syrup. Spoon the mixture over the apples. Bake for 25 minutes.

Cooking Tip:
Using liquid sweeteners for baking will help keep your cakes, cookies, muffins, etc. moist. You can expect cookies that use liquid instead of granular sweeteners to be chewy instead of crisp.

See glossary:
Agave syrup
Oats, rolled

1 SERVING = ²/₃ CUP/165 mL = 1 GRAIN + 1 FRUIT + ³/₄ NUT/SEED

PER SERVING			
calories-232	total fat-8 g	sodium-2 mg	iron-1.6 mg
protein-6 g	(saturated fat-1 g)	potassium-266 mg	calcium-30 mg
carbohydrates-38 g	fiber-5.6 g	vitamin A-8 RE	phosphorus-172 mg
	cholesterol-0 mg	vitamin C-8 mg	

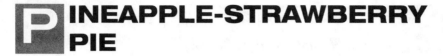INEAPPLE-STRAWBERRY PIE

Serves 10 (1 slice per serving)

CRUST

2 cups (500 mL) rolled oats
2 tablespoons (30 mL) ground flaxseed*
2 tablespoons (30 mL) canola oil
⅛ teaspoon (0.6 mL) salt (optional)
½ cup (125 mL) to ⅔ cup (165 mL) cold water

FILLING

3 cups (750 mL) peeled, cored, chopped fresh pineapple
5 tablespoons (75 mL) agar flakes
½ cup (125 mL) raw cashews
4 cups (1 L) hulled strawberries
½ teaspoon (2.5 mL) stevia

Preheat the oven to 375°F.

To make the crust, process the oats in a food processor or blender for about a minute or until the oats reach the texture of coarse flour.

Combine the oat flour, flaxseed, oil, salt, if using, and cold water in a medium bowl to form a sticky dough. With wet hands, press the dough into a 9-inch pie plate. Bake for 20 minutes. Remove from oven and set on a wire rack to cool.

To make the filling, process the pineapple in a food processor or blender until smooth. Place the pineapple purée in a medium saucepan with the agar flakes. Cook over medium heat for 5 minutes, stirring constantly. When the mixture begins to boil, lower the heat and simmer for 5 minutes.

While the pineapple mixture cooks, put the cashews in a food processor or blender and process until finely ground. Pour the pineapple mixture into the food processor or blender with the cashews. Add the strawberries and stevia, and process until smooth. Pour the purée into the pie shell and refrigerate several hours or overnight, until firm.

*To grind flaxseed, place in an electric mill, such as the type used to grind coffee beans, and pulse until finely ground, or crush using a heavy mortar and pestle.

Cooking Tip:

Use your food processor to chop nuts. Pulse it and keep an eye on them or they will become ground instead of chopped. A blender turns oatmeal into flour and grinds flax, sunflower, and sesame seeds into meal or ground seeds.

See glossary:

Agar flakes
Canola oil
Cashews, raw
Flaxseed
Oats, rolled
Stevia

1 SERVING = 1 SLICE = 1 GRAIN + 1 FRUIT + ¼ NUT/SEED

PER SERVING	total fat-7 g	sodium-7 mg	iron-1.7 mg
calories-166	(saturated fat-1 g)	potassium-239 mg	calcium-34 mg
protein-4 g	fiber-4.7 g	vitamin A-4 RE	phosphorus-123 mg
carbohydrates-23 g	cholesterol-0 mg	vitamin C-37 mg	

BRENDA'S DATE COOKIES

Makes 24 cookies (1 cookie per serving)

2 cups (500 mL) dates
½ cup (125 mL) water
1 tablespoon (15 mL) lemon juice
¼ cup (60 mL) canola oil
¼ cup (60 mL) soymilk
    or nonfat milk
1 teaspoon (5 mL) vanilla extract
1 tablespoon (15 mL) ground
    flaxseed*

¼ cup (60 mL) unsweetened
    applesauce or 1 grated apple
1 cup (250 mL) whole-wheat flour
2 teaspoons (10 mL) baking
    powder
½ teaspoon (2.5 mL) baking soda
½ teaspoon (2.5 mL) salt
½ cup (125 mL) walnuts, coarsely
    chopped

In a small saucepan over medium-high heat, cook the dates and water for about 5 minutes or until the dates are soft. Remove the dates and drain. Mash the dates with a potato masher.

Preheat the oven to 350°F.

In a large bowl, combine the lemon juice, oil, soymilk, vanilla, flaxseed, applesauce and dates. In a 2-cup measuring cup or small bowl, mix the flour, baking power, baking soda, and salt Add the dry ingredients to the wet ingredients and stir gently just until mixed. Fold in the walnuts.

Drop heaping teaspoonfuls of the dough onto a large, lightly oiled baking sheet. Bake for 15 minutes or until lightly browned. Remove the cookies from the oven, and let sit on the baking sheet 1 to 2 minutes to firm slightly. Remove the cookies to a wire rack to cool.

*To grind flaxseed, place in an electric mill, such as the type used to grind coffee beans, and pulse until finely ground, or crush using a heavy mortar and pestle.

See glossary:

Canola oil
Flaxseed
Soymilk

1 SERVING = 1 COOKIE = ½ GRAIN + ½ FRUIT + ¼ NUT/SEED

PER SERVING	total fat-4 g	sodium-102 mg	iron-0.5 mg
calories-98	(saturated fat-0 g)	potassium-136 mg	calcium-38 mg
protein-1 g	fiber-2.1 g	vitamin A-1 RE	phosphorus-72 mg
carbohydrates-15 g	cholesterol-0 mg	vitamin C-0 mg	

▌CED FRUIT CREAM

Serves 4 (½ cup/125 mL per serving)

2 frozen bananas
1 cup (250 mL) frozen strawberries
½ cup (125 mL) frozen blueberries
1 cup (250 mL) soymilk or nonfat milk
3 tablespoons (45 mL) frozen orange juice concentrate

In a food processor or blender, process all ingredients until smooth, adding more soymilk if needed to thin the mixture. Eat immediately or pack the mixture into a covered container and freeze for a firmer treat.

Cooking Tip:
Cut down your sugar consumption by replacing many sweeteners with fruit or alternative sweeteners. You will need to allow your taste buds time to adjust. Soon you will grow to appreciate the more subtle sweetness even more than the sugar buzz.

See glossary:
Soymilk

1 SERVING = ½ CUP/125 mL = 1 FRUIT + ½ LEGUME

PER SERVING	total fat-2 g	sodium-10 mg	iron-0.7 mg
calories-115	(saturated fat-0 g)	potassium-478 mg	calcium-16 mg
protein-3 g	fiber-3.6 g	vitamin A-13 RE	phosphorus-57 mg
carbohydrates-25 g	cholesterol-0 mg	vitamin C-47 mg	

TREATIE BALLS

Makes 20 balls (1 ball per serving)

½ cup (125 mL) sunflower seeds
3 tablespoons (45 mL) sesame seeds
½ cup (125 mL) walnuts
½ cup (125 mL) almond butter or cashew butter
¼ cup (60 mL) agave syrup or brown rice syrup
¼ cup (60 mL) carob powder
½ cup (125 mL) rolled oats
½ teaspoon (2.5 mL) vanilla extract

In a small, dry skillet over high heat, toast the sunflower seeds and walnuts, stirring often, taking care not to burn. Remove the seeds and nuts from the skillet and set aside to cool. Toast the sesame seeds in same skillet. Remove from the skillet and set aside to cool.

When cool, chop the seeds and nuts. Combine the chopped nuts and seeds in a mixing bowl with the nut butter, syrup, carob, oats, and vanilla. Mix well.

With wet hands, shape the mixture into 1-inch balls. Roll the balls in the toasted sesame seeds. Chill until ready to serve.

See glossary:

Agave syrup
Almond butter
Carob powder
Cashew butter
Oats, rolled

1 SERVING = 1 BALL = ½ NUT/SEED + ½ GRAIN

PER SERVING	total fat-8 g	sodium-8 mg	iron-0.9 mg
calories-110	(saturated fat- 1 g)	potassium-119 mg	calcium-33 mg
protein-3 g	fiber-1.4 g	vitamin A-1 RE	phosphorus-99 mg
carbohydrates-8 g	cholesterol-0 mg	vitamin C-0 mg	

MILLET PUDDING

Serves 4 (²⁄₃ cup/165 mL per serving)

⅓ cup (85 mL) millet
1¼ cups (310 mL) water
½ cup (125 mL) unsweetened pineapple juice
3 tablespoons (45 mL) raw cashews
1 teaspoon (5 mL) vanilla extract
⅛ teaspoon (0.6 mL) salt

In a small saucepan, bring the millet and water to a boil. Reduce the heat and simmer, covered, for 20 minutes or until the millet is tender and the water is absorbed.

While the millet cooks, combine the pineapple juice and cashews in a food processor or blender. Process until smooth. Add the hot millet along with the vanilla and salt and process briefly to mix.

Pour mixture into individual serving dishes and refrigerate until cool and firm. If desired, serve with fresh fruit.

Cooking Tip:		See glossary:
Before cooking millet, quinoa, or buckwheat, try toasting the grains in your cooking pot (dry roast, no oil) over medium heat. Stir until the grains are browned and aromatic. Then add your water and cover to cook. This imparts a nutty flavor to your finished grain.		Cashews, raw Millet

1 SERVING = ²⁄₃ CUP/165 mL = 1 GRAIN + ½ NUT/SEED

PER SERVING	total fat-4 g	sodium-67 mg	iron-1.1 mg
calories-164	(saturated fat-1 g)	potassium-139 mg	calcium-9 mg
protein-4 g	fiber-1.4 g	vitamin A-0 RE	phosphorus-127 mg
carbohydrates-28 g	cholesterol-0 mg	vitamin C-4 mg	

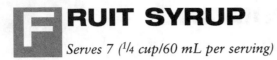

FRUIT SYRUP

Serves 7 (¹⁄₄ cup/60 mL per serving)

This syrup is equally delicious over a frozen dessert or pancakes and waffles.

4 cups (1 L) fresh berries
¹⁄₂ cup (125 mL) water or unsweetened apple juice concentrate
1 teaspoon (5 mL) cornstarch
2 tablespoons (30 mL) water

In a medium saucepan, crush the berries with a potato masher. Add the water or juice. Alternatively, the berries can be processed in a food processor or blender with the water or juice and then placed in the saucepan. Bring the berry mixture to a boil. Reduce the heat and simmer for several minutes.

While the berries simmer, dissolve the cornstarch in the water and add to the fruit mixture. Cook over low heat, stirring, until the sauce thickens.

Cooking Tip:

An easy way to measure liquid sweeteners that are thick and sticky is to measure the oil first—or rub just enough oil in the spoon or measuring cup to coat it. Then your sweetener will glide into your mixing bowl without sticking. You may need a rubber spatula to get it all out.

1 SERVING = ¹⁄₄ CUP/60 mL = ¹⁄₂ FRUIT

PER SERVING	total fat-0 g	sodium-3 mg	iron-0.2 mg
calories-37	(saturated fat-0 g)	potassium-108 mg	calcium-8 mg
protein-1 g	fiber-2.1 g	vitamin A- 5 RE	phosphorus-12 mg
carbohydrates-9 g	cholesterol-0 mg	vitamin C-30 mg	

CELERY SNACKS

Serves 9 (1 piece per serving)

1 California or Haas avocado,
  skinned, pitted
1 clove garlic, minced

2 teaspoons (10 mL) lemon juice
Pinch ground cumin
3 stalks celery

In a small bowl, mash together the avocado, garlic, lemon juice, and cumin. Spoon the mixture into the celery stalks. Cut the stalks into thirds and arrange on a serving plate.

1 SERVING = 1 PIECE = ½ NUT/SEED			
PER SERVING	total fat-3 g	sodium-18 mg	iron-0.3 mg
calories-39	(saturated fat-1 g)	potassium-186 mg	calcium-10 mg
protein-1 g	fiber-1.6 g	vitamin A-16 RE	phosphorus-14 mg
carbohydrates-2 g	cholesterol-0 mg	vitamin C-4 mg	

TAMARI ROASTED ALMONDS

Serves 12 (about 8 nuts per serving)

1 cup (250 mL) raw almonds
1 tablespoon (15 mL) tamari

Spread the almonds on a small baking sheet. Sprinkle the tamari over the almonds and stir.

Preheat the oven to 350°F. Bake the almonds for 10 minutes, stirring once. Continue baking 5 minutes more or until lightly browned. Cool completely before storing in an airtight jar.

See glossary:

  Tamari

1 SERVING = 8 NUTS = ½ NUT/SEED			
PER SERVING	total fat-6 g	sodium-73 mg	iron-0.4 mg
calories-64	(saturated fat-1 g)	potassium-82 mg	calcium-29 mg
protein-2 g	fiber-1.2 g	vitamin A-0 RE	phosphorus-58 mg
carbohydrates-2 g	cholesterol-0 mg	vitamin C-0 mg	

CUCUMBER-MINT DIP

Serves 6 (¹⁄₄ cup/60 mL per serving)

1 cucumber, seeded, chopped

1 cup (250 mL) yogurt, soy or nonfat plain

2 tablespoons (30 mL) flax oil or extra-virgin olive oil

2 tablespoons (30 mL) rice vinegar

¹⁄₂ cup (125 mL) fresh mint

1 teaspoon (5 mL) light miso

Combine all the ingredients in a food processor or blender, and process until smooth and creamy. Serve the dip with sliced vegetables or crackers if desired.

See glossary:

Extra-virgin olive oil
Flax oil
Miso
Rice vinegar
Soy yogurt

---

1 SERVING = ¹⁄₄ CUP/60 mL = ¹⁄₄ NUT/SEED

PER SERVING	total fat-3 g	sodium-14 mg	iron-0.2 mg
calories-31	(saturated fat-0 g)	potassium-67 mg	calcium-4 mg
protein-1 g	fiber-0.5 g	vitamin A-6 RE	phosphorus-16 mg
carbohydrates-1 g	cholesterol-0 mg	vitamin C-1 mg	

Rich source of omega-3 fatty acids if made with flax oil (providing at least 1 g per serving)

ROASTED GARLIC HUMMUS

Serves 8 (¹/₄ cup/60 mL per serving)

1 head garlic
2 cups (500 mL) cooked, drained garbanzo beans
¹/₄ cup (60 mL) bean stock or water
¹/₄ cup (60 mL) lemon juice
1 tablespoon (15 mL) tamari
3 tablespoons (45 mL) tahini
¹/₄ cup (60 mL) chopped fresh parsley

Preheat the oven to 350°F. Wrap the unpeeled head of garlic in aluminum foil. Roast in the oven for 45 minutes or until the cloves are soft.

When cool enough to handle, squeeze the cloves out of their skins and into a food processor or blender with the remaining ingredients. Process until smooth.

See glossary:

Garbanzo beans
Tahini
Tamari

Cooking Tip:

Cook extra beans so you can freeze some for a later meal. Freeze two to four cups at a time so you will be ready for a quick taco or tostada feast. All you will have to do is to defrost the beans and chop a few toppings.

1 SERVING = ¹/₄ CUP/60 mL = ¹/₂ LEGUME + ¹/₂ NUT/SEED

PER SERVING	total fat-4 g	sodium-134 mg	iron-1.5 mg
calories-103	(saturated fat-0 g)	potassium-167 mg	calcium-47 mg
protein-5 g	fiber-3 g	vitamin A-11 RE	phosphorus-116 mg
carbohydrates-14 g	cholesterol-0 g	vitamin C-6 mg	

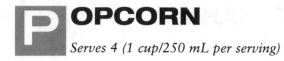

POPCORN

Serves 4 (1 cup/250 mL per serving)

A recipe for popcorn? Only to introduce you to the delicious, cheesy flavor of nutritional yeast flakes. This is the low-fat, nutritious alternative to cheese corn.

4 cups (1 L) freshly popped popcorn
2 tablespoons (30 mL) nutritional yeast flakes
1 tablespoon (15 mL) flax oil
Pinch of salt

Sprinkle the yeast, oil, and salt over the popcorn.

See glossary:

Flax oil
Nutritional yeast flakes

1 SERVING = 1 CUP/250 mL = 1 GRAIN			
PER SERVING	total fat-4 g	sodium-55 mg	iron-0.3 mg
calories-72	(saturated fat-0 g)	potassium-104 mg	calcium-3 mg
protein-3 g	fiber-1.2 g	vitamin A-2 RE	phosphorus-68 mg
carbohydrates-8 g	cholesterol-0 mg	vitamin C-0 mg	

Rich source of omega-3 fatty acids (providing at least 1 g per serving)

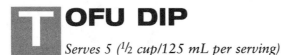OFU DIP

Serves 5 (½ cup/125 mL per serving)

1 tablespoon (15 mL) sesame seeds
½ pound (227 g) silken tofu
½ pound (227 g) firm tofu, crumbled
½ cup (125 mL) chopped green onion
½ cup (125 mL) diced celery
¼ cup (60 mL) minced fresh dill weed
3 tablespoons (45 mL) Nayonaise, Veganaise,
    or other mayonnaise-like spread
1 tablespoon (15 mL) apple cider vinegar
1 tablespoon (15 mL) tamari
½ tablespoon (7 mL) spicy mustard

In small dry skillet over high heat, toast the sesame seeds, stirring often, taking care not to burn. Remove from the skillet and set aside to cool.

In a food processor or blender, process the silken tofu until smooth. Set aside.

Combine the toasted sesame seeds, puréed silken tofu, and all the remaining ingredients in a serving bowl. Mix well. Serve with raw vegetables or spread on rice cakes or baked corn chips.

See glossary:

Nayonaise
Sesame seeds
Tamari
Tofu

---

1 SERVING = ½ CUP/125 mL = 1 LEGUME + ½ NUT/SEED

PER SERVING	total fat-11 g	sodium-310 mg	iron-10.1 mg
calories-171	(saturated fat-1 g)	potassium-295 mg	calcium-216 mg
protein-15 g	fiber-2.8 g	vitamin A-21 RE	phosphorus-195 mg
carbohydrates-6 g	cholesterol-0 mg	vitamin C-3 mg	

Glossary

Agar flakes—A clear, flavorless gelatin substitute made from seaweed. Available in both natural food stores and Asian markets.

Agave syrup—A liquid sweetener made from the agave cactus plant that is 90 percent fructose. You can substitute ½ cup (125 mL) agave syrup for 1 cup (250 mL) sugar in recipes (reduce liquid by ¼ cup; 60 mL).

Almond butter—A spreadable butter made from ground almonds.

Amaranth—An ancient grain cultivated primarily in South and Central America, but found in many parts of the world. Higher in protein than most grains, amaranth can be eaten as a whole grain or ground into flour and used to enrich bread and other baked goods. To prepare whole amaranth, cook 1 cup (250 mL) with 3 cups (750 mL) water for 20 to 30 minutes (yield: 3 cups; 750 mL).

Arrowroot—A starchy thickener that becomes clear when cooked. Can be used instead of cornstarch and needs to be dissolved in cold water before being added to hot liquids.

Arugula—A peppery salad green often called "rocket" and featured in Italian cuisine.

Balsamic vinegar—A rich, dark wine vinegar with delicious, complex flavor.

Barley—Barley is a chewy, versatile grain that is wonderful in soups and stews. It is one of the creamiest of all grains, and makes a delicious creamy pudding (similar to rice pudding). Hulled barley or pot barley has only the outer husk removed. It takes the longest to cook but it is the most nutritious. Scotch barley is husked and coarsely ground. Pearled barley, more commonly found in supermarkets, is hulled, has the bran removed, and has been steamed and polished. It takes the least time to cook. To prepare pearled barley, simmer 1 cup (250 mL) barley in 3 cups (750 mL) water for 40 to 50 minutes (yield: 3½ cups; 875 mL).

Barley flour—Flour ground from barley from which the hull and bran have been removed.

Barley malt—A sweetening syrup made from soaked, sprouted whole barley. See page 135 for information on cooking with barley malt.

Blackstrap molasses—A dark, strong-tasting liquid by-product of sugar refining. It contains significant amounts of minerals, calcium, and iron, more so than other types of molasses. See page 135 for information on cooking with blackstrap molasses.

Bok choy—A crunchy, mild Chinese cabbage. It has oblong white stems with pale green top leaves. Rich in calcium.

Bragg Liquid Aminos—A nonfermented, wheat-free substitute for soy sauce that has not been fermented. Available in natural food stores.

Brown rice—Rice in which only the husk has been removed. Brown rice will keep for about six months on the kitchen shelf, longer if refrigerated. To prepare, cook 1 cup (250 mL) brown rice with 2 cups (500 mL) water for 45 minutes (yield: 3 cups; 750 mL).

Brown rice syrup—A sweetening syrup made from brown rice, this is not a good substitute for sugar in recipes but can replace honey. See page 136 for information on cooking with brown rice syrup.

Buckwheat—Usually sold hulled or as groats (hulled and crushed), unless you are buying it for sprouting. When buckwheat groats are toasted they are called kasha. Buckwheat goes well with mushrooms, onions, cabbage, dill, and winter squash. To prepare buckwheat, simmer 1 cup (250 mL) buckwheat groats in 2½ cups (625 mL) water for 20 minutes (yield: 2½ cups; 625 mL).

Buckwheat flour—Made from ground buckwheat, technically not a grain, but a member of the rhubarb family; buckwheat is gluten-free, and therefore excellent for those who have wheat allergies.

Bulgur—Cracked wheat grains that have had the hulls removed. Can be prepared without cooking (unless it is the very coarse kind). Add 2 cups (500 mL) boiling water to 1 cup (250 mL) bulgur, and cover for 20 to 30 minutes.

Canola oil—A monounsaturated oil high in essential fatty acids, including omega-3.

Capers—Flower buds from a Mediterranean shrub, used as a condiment.

Carob powder—A caffeine-free substitute for cocoa, slightly sweeter, with a dark, earthy flavor.

Cashew butter—A spreadable butter made from ground raw cashews.

Cilantro—The fresh leaves of the coriander plant. It also is called Chinese or Mexican parsley.

Couscous—Crushed, steamed, and dried durum wheat, popular in Moroccan and other Middle Eastern dishes. Available in natural food stores.

Daikon—A very large, white Asian radishlike vegetable. It is very crunchy and sweet. Daikon can be used in stir-fries or salads.

Extra-virgin olive oil—A cold-pressed, unfiltered olive oil from the first pressing of the olives, where no chemicals are used to extract the oil. The color of the oil can vary according to the location and climate in which the olives were grown.

Fennel—A vegetable that looks similar to celery but has a slight licorice flavor.

Flaxseed (linseed)—A small brown seed that is high in omega-3 fatty acids (alpha-linolenic acid), soluble fiber, and the mineral boron. For maximum benefits, grind and use on cereals or in baking as an egg replacer. *Flax oil* is produced from flaxseed.

Garbanzo beans (chickpeas)—Round, light-brown beans with a nutty flavor. Traditionally used in Middle-Eastern dishes such as hummus and falafel.

Gingerroot—The whole root of the ginger plant. Slices of fresh gingerroot can be used in stir-frys and other vegetable dishes.

Gluten (seitan)—A meatlike food made from wheat protein. Gluten can be purchased as a powder to be mixed with water or as a ready-to-use product (called seitan) canned, refrigerated, or frozen. Gluten has a firm texture and neutral flavor. It easily picks up the flavors of the foods with which it is cooked.

Hempseed oil—Pressed from hempseeds, this oil is high in essential fatty acids.

Hoisin sauce—A thick brown sauce made from soybeans, garlic, chili peppers and other spices. Used in Chinese cooking.

Jalapeño pepper—A thick-skinned hot pepper, about two inches long. They are very often served sliced and pickled. Even the juice from fresh jalapeños is extremely hot and can burn your skin, so wear protective gloves if you plan to cut them for cooking or canning. Dried, smoked jalapeños, called chipotles, impact a wonderful earthy flavor and zest to beans and grains.

Kale—A delicious, nutritious green with dark green, ruffled leaves. Prepare by removing the thick stalk and sautéing or steaming the greens. Cook kale within a few days of purchasing to ensure the best flavor.

Kamut—An ancient wheat grain that has not been hybridized, so it retains a rich flavor. People with gluten allergies may find it easier to digest than regular wheat. Intact kamut berries are used as other wheat berries. Kamut berries are also ground into flour and used to make breads and pasta. To prepare, cook 1 cup (250 mL) kamut in 3 cups (750 mL) water for 50 to 60 minutes (yield: 3 cups; 750 mL).

Kasha—Buckwheat kernels which have been crushed and hulled, then roasted, yielding a nutty-flavored grain that's quick to cook up. Available in natural food stores and some supermarkets.

Legumes—Plant species that have seed pods that split along both sides when ripe. Some of the more common legumes used for human consumption are beans, lentils, peanuts, peas, and soybeans.

Marjoram—An herb with a delicate, oregano-like flavor.

Millet—A tiny, round, golden, gluten-free grain that becomes light and fluffy when cooked. Millet is a sticky grain, thus is excellent for use in patties and loaves. It is high in fiber and protein and has antifungal properties. Available in natural food stores and some supermarkets. To prepare, simmer 1 cup (250 mL) millet with 2½ cups (625 mL) water for 20 minutes (yield: 2½ cups; 625 ml).

Miso—A salty paste made from cooked, aged soybeans and sometimes grains such as barley and rice. Thick and spreadable, it's used for flavoring and soup bases. It comes in several varieties; darker varieties tend to be stronger flavored and saltier than lighter varieties. Available in natural food stores and some Asian grocery stores.

Mustard greens—A nutritious green with very ruffled leaves and a characteristic pungent flavor of mustard. They are at their best in the cooler fall and winter months. Mustard leaves can be sautéed or steamed.

Nutritional yeast flakes—A dietary supplement and condiment, rich in B vitamins, that has a distinct cheeselike flavor and a pleasant aroma. Although there are many brands of nutritional yeast flakes, Red Star makes a variety that is particularly good for vegans (T6635+), because it is a reliable source of vitamin B_{12}. Nutritional yeast is not leavening yeast used in making bread. It is available in natural food stores and some grocery stores.

Oats—One of the most nutritious grains, oats come in many forms besides the *rolled oats* used to make oatmeal cereal. *Oat groats* (or steel-cut or Irish oats) are whole oats which have been cleaned, hulled, and sometimes cut into several pieces so they can be cooked and eaten similar to rice. They make a tasty morning cereal. *Oat flour* is usually made by grinding oat groats, but you can also make small amounts at home by pulverizing rolled oats in a dry blender or coffee grinder. Oat groats, oat flour, and rolled oats can also be used as thickeners for sauces, loaves, and stuffing as well as added to cakes, breads, muffins, pancakes, and, of course, granola. *Oat bran* is high in soluble fiber and can be used as part of a high-fiber diet to reduce cholesterol levels. To prepare oat groats as a whole grain (similar to how you would serve rice), simmer 1 cup (250 mL) with 3 cups (750 mL) water for 1 hour, or soak overnight to lessen cooking time (yield: 2½ cups; 625 mL).

Polenta—A creamy cooked dish made from coarse cornmeal, similar in consistency to southern grits or Cream of Wheat. Often it is allowed to cool, then cut into pieces and served with a variety of pasta sauces.

Pulses—Dried seeds of legumes.

Quinoa (pronounced keen-wa)—An ancient grain of the Incas, quinoa is nicknamed the "supergrain" because it contains more high-quality protein than any other grain. This round, sand-colored, quick-cooking grain has a light texture and a mild, nutty taste. It is very low in gluten, which makes it a good substitute for those who have wheat allergies. To prepare, simmer 1 cup (250 mL) quinoa with 2 cups (500 mL) water for 15 minutes (yield: 3 cups; 750 mL). Wash well before cooking to remove the natural, strong-tasting resin that coats the grain.

Raw nuts—Any nuts that have not been roasted or toasted. Raw nuts should be stored in the refrigerator for up to a month, or up to six months in the freezer, to prevent them from becoming rancid.

Raw sugar—Coarse, minimally refined sugar made from sugar cane or sugar beets.

Rice flour—Ground from white rice, rice flour can be used to replace some or all of the wheat flour in certain recipes.

Rice milk—A grain beverage similar in appearance to cow's milk, made by puréeing rice and water, then straining it. Although it can be used by those who have a sensitivity to cow's milk or soymilk, it is lower in protein, calcium, and fat.

Rice vinegar—A mild, slightly sweet vinegar made from fermented rice. A staple in Japanese cooking, rice vinegar can be found in natural food stores and Asian groceries.

Rye—A hearty plant, used as a green cover crop over the winter because it can withstand freezing weather. It has a strong flavor and can be used whole, cracked, or as flour, usually in breads. To prepare as a whole grain, simmer 1 cup (250 mL) rye berries (unhulled rye) in 3 cups (750 mL) water for 1 hour, or soak overnight to lessen cooking time (yield: 3 cups; 750 mL).

Rye flour—Rye flour is usually combined with other flours in baked goods. On its own, it will make a very dense, heavy bread. *Dark rye flour* is used to make dark rye bread with its rich flavor; it can be found in many natural food stores and some supermarkets.

Savory (summer and winter)—An excellent herb to use with bean dishes, imparting a flavor somewhere between thyme and mint. Summer savory is slightly milder than winter savory.

Soy flour—A high-protein flour made from grinding whole soybeans. Because it is gluten-free, it cannot replace wheat flour in baking, but you can usually replace ¼ cup (60 mL) wheat flour with an equal amount of soy flour to increase the protein content of the recipe.

Soymilk—A nondairy milky liquid made from grinding soybeans, then simmering them in water and straining. Soymilk can be used in almost any recipe calling for cow's milk with similar results, including to make *soy yogurt*. Plain, unflavored soymilk is the best choice for cooking and baking; the many flavored soymilks now available at natural food stores and some supermarkets are favored by many people for drinking, either right out of the carton or in smoothies or shakes. Many soymilks are now fortified with calcium and other nutrients.

Spelt—An ancient grain similar to wheat. It may be easier for people with gluten allergies to digest than wheat. To prepare, simmer 1 cup (250 mL) spelt with 3 cups (750 mL) water for 50 to 60 minutes (yield: 3 cups; 750 mL).

Stevia—An herb whose leaves are ground and dried or extracted into a white powder to use as a natural alternative sweetener. The strength of the stevia you find will depend on the form it is in; the extract has much more sweetening power than dried, ground stevia. It is a popular sweetening alternative in Japan and South America.

Tahini—A thick, smooth paste made of either raw or toasted, ground sesame seeds. Available in natural food stores, Middle Eastern or gourmet groceries, and some supermarkets. Rich in calcium.

Tamari—A type of soy sauce naturally fermented from soybeans. Its rich, complex flavor is worth the extra cost compared to varieties of soy sauce found on most supermarket shelves.

Tempeh—A high-protein, highly digestible, cultured food made from soybeans and sometimes grains. Available in Asian grocery stores and natural food stores.

Toasted sesame oil—This dark, nutty oil imparts a rich, delicious flavor with only a few drops, so you only need a little; a great choice for use in a low-fat menu.

Tofu (soybean curd)—A highly versatile soy product made from the milk of soybeans and coagulated with nigari or calcium salts. Available in many textures from soft to extra-firm. Medium-firm tofu, when made with calcium salts, provides an excellent source of calcium, while extra-firm tofu made with nigari provides higher levels of zinc and iron. Herbed tofu is an excellent option. Flavored tofu is especially convenient. It requires no cooking or flavoring and can be sliced and eaten like cheese, or used in sandwiches, salads and stir-fries. Many food products are made from tofu including nondairy milks, soy cheese, and meat substitutes.

Turmeric—A pungent, yellow spice often used in Indian cooking and reputed to have health-giving qualities.

Selected References

Chapter 1

Chen, Y. D. and G. M. Reaven. "Insulin resistance and atherosclerosis." *Diabetes Reviews* 5 (1997): 331-42.

Gohil, B. C., et al. "Hypothalmic–pituitary–adrenal axis function and the metabolic syndrome X of obesity." *CNS Spectrums* 6, no. 7 (2001): 581-89.

Reaven, G. M. "Pathophysiology of insulin resistance in human disease." *Physiological Review* 75 (1995): 473-86.

Reaven, G. M. "Role of insulin resistance in human disease." *Diabetes* 37 (1988): 1595-1607.

Reaven, G. M., H. Lithell, and L. Landsberg. "Hypertension and associated metabolic abnormalities—the role of insulin resistance and the sympatholadrenal system." *New England Journal of Medicine* 334 (1996): 374-81.

Reaven, Gerarld, T. Kristen Strom, and B. Fox. *Syndrome X*. New York, NY: Simon and Schuster, 2000.

Rexrode, K. M. and J. E. Manson. "Postmenopausal hormone therapy and quality of life, no cause for celebration." *New England Journal of Medicine* 287 (2002): 642-43.

Chapter 2

American Diabetes Association; Franz, M. J., et al. "Evidence-based nutrition principles and recommendations for the treatment and prevention of diabetes and related complications." *Diabetes Care* 25 (2002): 148-98.

Anderson, R. A., N. Cheng, N.A. Bryden, et al. "Beneficial effects of chromium for people with diabetes." *Diabetes* 46 (1997): 1786–91.

Anderson, J. W. "Nutrition management of diabetes mellitus," in *Modern Nutrition in Health and Disease*, 7th ed. Ed. By Shils, M.E. et al. New York, 1988.

Anderson, J. W,. et al. "Hypocholesterolemic effects of high fibre diets rich in water-soluble plant fibers." *Journal of the Canadian Dietetic Association* 45 (1984): 140-49.

Barnard, R. J., et al. "Long-term use of a high-complex-carbohydrate, high-fiber, low-fat diet and exercise in the treatment of NIDDM patients." *Diabetes Care* 6 (1983): 268-73.

Chandalia, M., et al. "Beneficial effects of a high dietary fiber intake in patients with type 2 diabetes.: *New England Journal of Medicine* 342 (2000): 1392–98.

Cheng, N., X. Zhu, Shi, H. et al. "Follow-up survey of people in China with type 2 diabetes mellitus consuming supplemental chromium." *Journal of Trace Elements Exploratory Medicine* 12 (1999): 55–60.

Christiansen, E., S. Schnider, B. Palmvig, et al. "Intake of a diet high in trans monounsaturated fatty acids or saturated fatty acids. Effects on postprandial insulinemia and glycemia in obese patients with NIDDM." *Diabetes Care* 20 no. 5 (1997): 881-87.

Coulston, A. M., et al. "Persistence of hypertriglyceridemic effect of low-fat high-carbohydrate diets in NIDDM patients." *Diabetes Care* 12 (1989): 94–101.

Cusi, K., et al. "Vanadyl sulfate improves hepatic and muscle insulin sensitivity in type 2 diabetes." *Journal of Clinical Endocrinology Metabolism* 86 no. 3 (March 2001): 1410-17.

de Lorgeril, M., M. P. Salen, J. Delaye. "Effect of a Mediterranean type of diet on the rate of cardiovascular complications in patients with coronary artery disease." *Journal of the American College of Cardiology* 28 no. 5 (1996): 1103-08.

de Lorgeril, M., M. P. Salen, J. L. Martin, et al. "Mediterranean diet, traditional risk factors, and the rate of cardiovascular complications after myocardial infarction: final report of the Lyon Diet Heart Study." *Circulation* 99 (February 1999): 779-85.

Esselstyn, C. B., Jr. "Updating a 12-year experience with arrest and reversal therapy of coronary heart disease." *American Journal of Cardiology* 84 no. 3 (August 1999): 339-41.

Feskens, E. J., D. Kromhout. "Habitual dietary intake and glucose tolerance in euglycaemic men: the Zutphen Study." *International Journal of Epidemiology* 19 (1990): 953-59.

Feskens, E. J. M., S. M. Virtanen, L. Räsänen, et al. "Dietary factors determining diabetes and impaired glucose tolerance. A 20-year follow-up of the Finnish and Dutch cohorts of the Seven Countries Study." *Diabetes Care* 18 (1995): 1104-12.

Foster-Powell, K. and Brand Miller, J. "International tables of glycemic index." *American Journal of Clinical Nutrition* 62 (1995): 8715-935.

Garg, A., et al. "Effects of varying carbohydrate content of diet in patients with non-insulin dependent diabetes mellitus." *Journal of the American Medical Association* 271 (1994): 1421–28.

Guthrie, D. and Guthrie R. *The Diabetes Sourcebook*. Los Angeles: Lowell House, 1999.

Hollenbeck, C. B. and Coulston, A.M. "Effects of dietary carbohydrate and fat intake on glucose and lipoprotein metabolism in individuals with diabetes mellitus." *Diabetes Care* 14 no. 9 (September 1991): 774-85.

Hollenbeck, C. B., et al. "The effects of variations in percent of naturally occurring complex and simple carbohydrates on plasma glucose and insulin response in individuals with non-insulin-dependent diabetes mellitus." *Diabetes* 34 (1985): 151–55.

Hu, F. B., R. M. van Dam, S. Liu. "Diet and risk of Type II diabetes: the role of types of fat and carbohydrate." *Diabetologia* 44 no. 7 (July 2001): 805-17.

Jenkins, D. J. "Metabolic advantages of spreading the nutrient load: effects of increased meal frequency in non-insulin dependent diabetes." *American Journal of Clinical Nutrition* 55 (1992): 461-67.

Jenkins, D. J. "Nibbling versus gorging: metabolic advantages of increased meal frequency." *New England Journal of Medicine* 321: 949-49.

Kao, W. H., et al. "Serum and dietary magnesium and the risk for type 2 diabetes mellitus: the Atherosclerosis Risk in Communities Study." *Archives of Internal Medicine* 159 no. 18 (1999): 2151-59.

Kiehm, T. G., J. W. Anderson, K. Ward. "Beneficial effects of a high carbohydrate, high fiber diet on hyperglycemic diabetic men." *American Journal of Clinical Nutrition* 29 (1976): 895-99.

Lichtenstein, A. H.; U. S. Schwab. "Relationship of dietary fat to glucose metabolism." *Atherosclerosis* 150 (2000): 227-43.

Marshall, J. A.; D. H. Bessesen, R. F. Hamman. "High saturated fat and low starch and fibre are associated with hyperinsulinemia in a non-diabetic population: The San Luis Valley Diabetes Study." *Diabetologia* 40 (1997): 430-38.

Marshall, J. A., R. F. Hamman, J. Baxter. "High-fat, low-carbohydrate diet and the etiology of non-insulin-dependent diabetes mellitus: The San Luis Valley Diabetes Study." *American Journal of Epidemiology* 134 (1991): 590-603.

Marshall, J. A.; S. Hoag, S. Shetterly, et al. "Dietary fat predicts conversion from impaired glucose tolerance to NIDDM: The San Luis Valley Diabetes Study." *Diabetes Care* 17 (1994): 50-56.

McDougall, J. "Rapid reduction of serum cholesterol and blood pressure by a twelve-day, very-low-fat, strictly vegetarian diet." *Journal of the American College of Nutrition* 14 no. 5 (October 1995): 491-96.

Nicholson, A., et al. "Toward improved management of NIDDM: A randomized, controlled, pilot intervention using a lowfat vegetarian diet." *Preventive Medicine* 29 (1999): 87-91.

O'Dea, K., et al. "The effects of diet differing in fat, carbohydrate, and fiber on carbohydrate and lipid metabolism in type II diabetes." *Journal of the American Dietetic Association* 89 no. 8 (August 1989): 1076-86.

Ornish D., et al. "Can lifestyle changes reverse coronary heart disease?" *Lancet 336 (1990)*: 129-33.

Ornish D., L. W. Scherwitz, J. H. Billings, et al. "Intensive lifestyle changes for reversal of coronary heart disease." *Journal of the American Medical Association* 280 no. 23 (December 1998): 2001-07.

Pan, D. A., S. Lillioja, A. D. Kriketos, et al. "Skeletal muscle triglyceride levels are inversely related to insulin action." *Diabetes* 46 (1997): 983-88.

Shintani, T,. et al. "Obesity and cardiovascular risk intervention through the ad libitum feeding of traditional Hawaiian diet." *American Journal of Clinical Nutrition* 53 no. 6 (June 1991): 1647S-51S.

Singh, I. "Low fat diet and therapeutic doses of insulin in diabetes mellitus." *Lancet* 1 (1955): 422-25.

Stone, D. B., et al. "The prolonged effects of a low cholesterol, high carbohydrate diet upon the serum lipids in diabetic patients." *Diabetes* 12 (1963): 127-32.

Storlien, L. H., L. A. Baur, A. D. Kriketos, et al. "Dietary fats and insulin action." *Diabetologia* 39 (1996): 621-31.

Thompson, K.H., et al. "Vanadium compounds as insulin mimetics." *Chemistry Review* 99 (1999): 2561-71.

Vessby, B., I. B. Gustafsson, J. Boberg, et al. "Substituting polyunsaturated for saturated fat as a single change in a Swedish diet: effects on serum lipoprotein metabolism and glucose tolerance in patients with hyperlipoproteinaemia." *European Journal of Clinical Investigation* 10 (1980): 193-202.

Vessby, B., M. Uusitupa, K. Hermansen, et al. "Substituting dietary saturated for monounsaturated fat impairs insulin sensitivity in healthy men and women: the KANWU study." *Diabetologia* 44 (2001): 312-19.

World Health Organization. "The scientific basis for diet, nutrition and the prevention of cancer." Background paper for the Joint WHO/FAO Expert Consultation on diet, nutrition and the prevention of chronic diseases, Geneva, 28 January–1 February 2002.

Chapter 3

Ågren, J., M. Törmälä, M. Nenonen, et al. "Fatty acid composition of erythrocyte, platelet, and serum lipids in strict vegans." *Lipids* 30 (1995): 365-69.

Allison, D. B., S. K. Egan, L. M. Barraj, et al. "Estimated intakes of trans fatty and other fatty acids in the US population." *Journal of the American Dietetic Association* 99 no. 2 (1999): 166-74.

American Diabetes Association. "Evidence-based nutrition principles and rec-ommendations for the treatment and prevention of diabetes and related complications." *Diabetes Care* 25 (2002):148-98.

American Diabetes Association. "Nutrition recommendations and principles for people with diabetes mellitus." *Diabetes Care* 17 (1994): 519-22.

American Dietetic Association. "Position of the American Dietetic Associa-tion: Vegetarian Diets." *Journal of the American Dietetic Association* 97 no. 11 (1997): 1317-132.

Anderson, J. W., B. M. Smith and J. Gustasson. "The practicality of high fibre diets." *American Journal of Clinical Nutrition* 59 (1994): 1242S-47S.

Barnard, R. J. "Effects of life-style modification of serum lipids." *Archives of Internal Medicine* 151 (1991): 1389-94.

Block, A. and Thompson, C. A. "Position of the American Dietetic Associa-tion: phytochemicals and functional foods." *Journal of the American Dietetic Association* 95 (1995): 493-96.

Carlson, E. A. "Comparative evaluation of vegan, vegetarian, and omnivore diets." *Journal of Plant Foods* 6 (1985): 89-100.

Conquer, J. A. and Holub, B. J. "Supplementation with an algae source of docosahexaenoic acid increases (n-3) fatty acid status and alters selected risk factors for heart disease in vegetarian subjects." *Journal of Nutrition* 126 (1996): 3032-39.

Craig, W. J. *Nutrition and Wellness. A vegetarian way to better health.* Berrien Springs, Michigan: Golden Harvest Books, 1999.

Craig, W. J. "Phytochemicals: Guardians of our health." *Issues in Vegetarian Dietetics* 5 no. 3 (Spring 1996): 1, 6-8.

Craig, W. J. *The Use and Safety of Common Herbs and Herbal Teas*, 2nd edition. Berrien Springs, Michigan: Golden Harvest Books, 1996.

Crane, M. G., R. Zielinski, R. Aloia. "Cis and trans fats in omnivores, lacto-ovo vegetarians and vegans." *American Journal of Clinical Nutrition* 48 (1988): 920 (abstr P2).

Cummings, J. H. and Macfarlane, G. T. "The control and consequences of bacterial fermentation in the human colon." *Journal of Applied Bacteriology* 70 (1991): 443-59.

Cunnane, S. C., S. Ganguli, C. Menard, et al. "High alpha-linolenic acid flaxseed: some nutritional properties in humans." *British Journal of Nutrition* 69 (1993): 443-53.

Davies, G. J. "Dietary fibre intakes of individuals with different eating pat-terns." *Human Nutrition Applied Nutrition* 39 no. 2 (April 1985): 139-48.

Davis, B. and Melina, V. *Becoming Vegan.* Summertown, TN: Book Publishing Co., 2000.

Food and Nutrition Board Institute of Medicine. *Dietary Reference Intakes.* Washington DC.: National Academy Press. Available online at: http://www.nap.edu/index.html

Foster-powell, K. and Brand, Miller J. "International tables of glycemic index." *American Journal of Clinical Nutrition* 62 (1995): 871S-93S.

Fraser, G. E. "Diet and coronary heart disease; beyond dietary fats and low-density-lipoprotein cholesterol." *American Journal of Clinical Nutrition* 59 no. 5 (May 1994): 1117S-23S.

Gartner, C., W. Stahl, H. Sies. "Lycopene is more bioavailable from tomato paste than from fresh tomatoes." *American Journal of Clinical Nutrition* 66 (1997): 116-22.

Groff, J. L., S. S. Gropper, S. M. Hunt. *Advanced Nutrition and Human Metabolism.* St Paul, MN: West Publishing Co, 1995.

Hasler, C. M. "Functional Foods: Their role in disease prevention and health promotion." *Food Technology* 52 no.11 (1998): 63-70.

Holt, S., J. C. Brand Miller, P. Petcoz. "Relationships between satiety and plasma glucose and insulin responses to foods." Proceedings of the Nutrition Society of Australia 20 (1996): 177.

Holub, B. J. and Celi, B. "Relationships of alpha-linolenic acid to platelet fatty acid composition and trans content of cholesterol-free foods." *Nutrition* 8 no. 2 (March/April 1992): 136-38.

Hu, F. B. and Stampfer, M. J. "Nut consumption and risk of coronary heart disease: a review of epidemiologic evidence." *Current Atherosclerosis Reports* 1 (1999): 205-10.

Jacobs, D. R., L. Slavin, and L. Marquart. "Whole grain intake and cancer; A review of the literature." *Nutrition and Cancer* 24 (1995): 221-29.

Kies, C. V. "Mineral utilization of vegetarians: Impact of variation in fat intake." *American Journal of Clinical Nutrition* 48 (1988): 884-87.

Kitts, D. D. "Bioactive substances in food." *Canadian Journal of Physiological Pharmacology* 72 (1993): 423-34.

Kontessis, P. A. "Renal, metabolic, and hormonal responses to proteins of different origin in normotensive, nonproteinuric type I diabetic patients." *Diabetes Care* 18 no. 9 (September 1995): 1233.

Krajcovicova-Kudlackova, M., R. Simoncic, A. Bederova, et al. "Plasma fatty acid profile and alternative nutrition." *Annals of Nutritional Metabolics* 41 no. 6 (1997): 365-70.

Li, D., et al. "The association of diet and thrombotic risk factors in healthy male vegetarians and meat-eaters." *European Journal of Clinical Nutrition* 53 (1999): 612-19.

Livesey, G. "Metabolizable energy of macronutrients." *American Journal of Clinical Nutrition* 62 (1995): 1135S-42S.

Loma Linda University. "Protein in vegetarian diets." *Vegetarian Health Letter* 1 no. 7 (1998): 1-3. email: vegletter@sph.llu.edu

Loma Linda University. "Sodium and health." *Vegetarian Nutrition Health Letter* 3 no. 2 (2000); 1-3. email: vegletter@sph.llu.edu

Mackay, S. and Ball, M. J. "Do beans and oatbran add to the effectivness of a low fat diet?" *European Journal of Clinical Nutrition* 46 (1992): 641-48.

Mann, J. I. "Dietary determinants of ischemic heart disease in health conscious individuals." *Heart* 78 no. 5 (November 1997): 450-55.

Marwick, C. "Learning how phytochemicals help fight disease." *Journal of the American Medical Association* 274 no. 17 (1995): 1328-31.

McCarron, D. "The dietary guideline for sodium: should we shake it up? Yes!" *American Journal of Clinical Nutrition* 71 (2000): 1013-19.

McNutt, K. "Medicinals in foods." *Nutrition Today* 30 (1995): 218-22.

Melina, V., Davis, B. and Harrison, V. *Becoming Vegetarian.* Summertown, TN: Book Publishing Co., 1995.

Messina, M. and Erdman, J. W., eds. "Second International Symposium on the role of soy in preventing and treating chronic disease." *American Journal of Clinical Nutrition* 68 no. 6S (1998): 1329S-1515.

Messina, M. and Messina, V. *The Dietitians Guide to Vegetarian Diets.* Gathersburg MD: Aspen Publishers, 1996.

Mezzano, D. and Beilin, L. J. "Vegetarian and other complex diets, fats, fiber, and hypertension." *American Journal of Clinical Nutrition* 59 no. 5 (May 1994): 1130S-35S.

Millward, J. "Meat or wheat for the next millenium? The nutritional value of plant-based diets in relation to human amino acid and protein requirements." *Proceedings of the Nutrition Society* 58 (1999): 249-60.

Milner, J. A. "Nonnutritive Components in Foods as Modifiers of the Cancer Process." In: *Preventive Nutrition: The Comprehensive Guide for Health Professionals.* Edited by Bendich, A. and Deckelbaum, R. J. Totowa NJ: Humana Press Inc.

Pennington, J. A. *Bowes and Church's Food Values of Portions Commonly Used.* 16th ed. Philadelphia: JB Lippincott Co, 1994.

Rainey, C. and Nyquist, L. "Nuts—Nutrition and health benefits of daily use." *Nutrition Today* 32 no. 4 (July/August 1997): 157-63.

Report of Joint FAO/WHO. "Expert consultation, protein quality evaluation, food and nutrition paper" 51, FAO of the United Nations, 1991

Sabaté, J., G. E. Fraser, K. Burke, et al. "Effects of walnuts on serum lipid levels and blood pressure in normal men." *New England Journal of Medicine* 328 (1993): 603-07.

Salmeron, J., F. B. Hu, J. E. Manson, et al. "Dietary fat intake and risk of type 2 diabetes in women." *American Journal of Clinical Nutrition* 73 no. 6 (June 2001): 1019-26.

Simopoulos, A. P. "Essential fatty acids in health and chronic disease." *American Journal of Clinical Nutrition* 70 no. 3 (September 1999): 560S-69S.

Simopoulos, A. P. and Robinson, J. *The Omega Plan.* New York, NY: Harper Collins Publishers, 1998.

Sola, R., A. E. Ville, J. L. Richard, et al. "Oleic acid rich diet protects against the oxidative modification of high density lipoproteins." *Free Radicals in Biological Medicine* 22 no. 6 (1997): 1037-45.

The Joint FAO/WHO Expert Consultation on Carbohydrates in Human Nutrition, April 1997. http://www.fao.org/WAICENT/FAOINFO/ECO-NOMIC/ESN/Carbweb/carbo.pfd

The Report of the Scientific Review Committee. Nutrition Recommendations. Health and Welfare Canada, 1990

Third International Congress on Vegetarian Nutrition. *American Journal of Clinical Nutrition* 70 supplement (1999): (entire issue)

Thompson, L. U. "Antioxidants and hormone-mediated health benefits of whole grains." *Critical Review of Food Science Nutrition* 34 (1994): 473-97.

Thompson, L. U. "Potential health benefits of whole grains and their components." *Contemporary Nutrition* 17 no. 6 (1992): 1-2.

Turley, M. L., C. M. Skeaff, J. I. Mann, et al. "The effect of a low-fat, high-carbohydrate diet on serum high density lipoprotein cholesterol and triglyceride." *European Journal of Clinical Nutrition* 52 no. 10 (October 1998): 728-32.

United States Department of Agriculture. *Agriculture Fact Book 1998*. Office of Communications. www.usda.gov/news/pubs/fbook98/content.htm

USDA Nutrient Database for Standard Reference: http://www.nal.usda.gov/fnic/cgi-bin/nut_search.pl

Vaisey-Genser, M. *Flaxseed: Health, Nutrition and Functionality*. Winnipeg Canada: The Flax Council of Canada.

Viola, P. *Olive Oil and Health*. Spain: International Olive Oil Council, 1997.

World Cancer Research Fund in Association with American Institute of Cancer Research. *Food, Nutrition and the Prevention of Cancer: a Global Perspective*. Menasha WI: Banta Book Group, 1997.

World Health Organization and FAO Joint Consultation. "Fats and Oils in Human Nutrition." *Nutritional Review* (1994): 202-05.

World Health Organization Study Group on Diet, Nutrition and the Prevention of Non-communicable Diseases. "Diet, Nutrition and the Prevention of Chronic Diseases." Geneva, Switzerland: Technical Report Series No. 797. World Health Organization, 1991.

World Health Organization. Background paper for the Joint WHO/FAO Expert Consultation on diet, nutrition and the prevention of chronic diseases. Annex 3: "The scientific basis for diet, nutrition and the prevention of Type 2 diabetes." Geneva, Switzerland. 28 January–1 February 2002.

Chapter 4

Alfieri, M., J. Pomerleau, D. N. Grace. "A comparison of fat intake of normal weight, moderately obese and severely obese subjects." *Obesity Surgery* 7 no. 1 (1997): 9-15.

Allison, D. B., et al. "Annual deaths attributable to obesity in the United States." *Journal of the American Dietetic Association* 282 (1999): 1530-38.

American Dietetic Association. "Position of the American Dietetic Association: weight management." *Journal of the American Dietetic Association* 9 no. 1 (1997): 71-74.

American Dietetic Association. "Send fat diets packing." January 1999. From the ADA web site www.eatright.org.

Appleby, P. N., M. Thorogood, J. I. Mann, et al. "Low body mass index in non meat eaters: the possible roles of animal fat, dietary fibre and alcohol." *International Journal of Obesity Related Metabolic Disorders* 22 no. 5 (1998): 454-60.

Atkins, R. C. *Dr. Atkins' New Diet Revolution.* New York: M. Evans & Co., 1992.

Baer, D. J., W. V. Rumpler, C. W. Miles, et al. "Dietary fiber decreases the metabolizable energy content and nutrient digestibility of mixed diets fed to humans." *Journal of Nutrition* 127 no. 4 (1997): 579-86.

Blackburn, G. "Effect of degree of weight loss on health benefits." *Obesity Research* 3 no. 2 (1995): 211s-16s.

Blundell, J.E., C. L. Lawton, A. J. Hill. "Mechanisms of appetite control and their abnormalities in obese patients." *Hormone Research* 39 no. 3 (1993): 72-76.

Bonham, G. S. and Brock, D. B. "The relationship of diabetes with race, sex, and obesity." *American Journal of Clinical Nutrition* 41 (1985): 776-83.

Bray, G. A. "Complications of obesity". *Annals of Internal Medicine* 103 no. 6 (1985): 1052-62.

Brown, et al. *State of the World 2000.* Washington D. C.: Worldwatch Institute, 1999. www.worldwatch.org

Brownell, K. D. "Personal responsibility and control over our bodies: When expectation exceeds reality." *Health Psychology* 10 no. 5 (1991): 303-10.

Chan, J. M., et al. "Obesity, fat distribution, and weight gain as risk factors for clinical diabetes in men." *Diabetes Care* 17 (1994): 961-69.

Cheuvront, S. N. "The zone diet and athletic performance." *Sports Medicine* 27 no. 4 (April 1999): 213-28.

Colditz, G. A., et al. "Weight gain as a risk factor for clinical diabetes mellitus in women." *Annals of Internal Medicine* 122 (1995): 481-86.

Cordero-MacIntryre, Z. "Obesity and body fat distribution: A role for vegetarian diets?" Fourth International Congress on Vegetarian Nutrition. Loma Linda University, April, 2002.

Daly, M. E., C. Vale, M. Walker, et al. "Dietary carbohydrates and insulin sensitivity: a review of the evidence and clinical implications." *American Journal of Clinical Nutrition* 66 no. 5 (1997): 1072.

Delargy, H. J., K. R. O'Sullivan, R. J. Fletcher, et al. "Effects of amount and type of dietary fibre (soluble and insoluble) on short-term control of appetite." *International Journal of Food Science and Nutrition* 48, no. 1 (1997): 67-77.

Després, J. P. "Abdominal obesity as important component of insulin-resistance syndrome." *Nutrition* 9 (1993): 452-59.

Eades, M. R. *Protein Power.* New York: Bantam Books, 1996.

Foreyt, J. P. and Goodrick, K. "Weight management without dieting." *Nutrition Today* (March/April 1993): 4-9.

Harvey-Berino, J. "The efficacy of dietary fat vs. total energy restriction for weight loss." *Obesity Research* 6 no. 3 (1998): 202-07.

Health and Welfare Canada. "Canadian Guidelines for Healthy Weights." Report of an Expert Group convened by Health Promotion Directorate, Health Services and Promotion Branch. Ottawa, Canada: Minister of Supply and Services, 1988.

Institute of Medicine. *Weighing the Options: Criteria for Evaluating Weight-Management Programs.* Washington, DC: National Academy Press, 1995.

Khouzam, Skelton N. and Skelton W. "Medical implications of obesity." *Postgraduate Medicine* 92 no. 1 (1992): 151-62.

Kuczmarski, R. J., M. D. Carrol, K. M. Flegal, et al. "Varying body mass index cutoff points to describe overweight prevalence among U.S. adults: NHANES III (1988-1994)." *Obesity Research* 5 (1997): 542.

Levin, N., J. Rattan, and T. Gilat. "Energy intake and body weight in ovo-lacto vegetarians." *Journal of Clinical Gastroenterology* 8 no. 4 (1986): 451-53.

Ludwig, D. S., J. A. Majzoub, A. Al-Zahrani, et al. "High glycemic index foods, overeating, and obestiy." *Pediatrics* 103 no. 3 (1999): E26.

Marniemi, J., A. Seppanen, P. Hakala, P. "Long-term effects on lipid metabolism of weight reduction on lactovegetarian and mixed diet." *International Journal of Obesity* 14 no. 2 (1990): 113-25.

McNutt, K. "Fat traps, tips and tricks." *Nutrition Today* (May/June 1992): 47-49.

Mokhad, A. H., et al. "The spread of the obesity epidemic in the United States, 1991-1998." *Journal of the American Medical Association* 282 (1999): 1519-22.

National Institutes of Health. "Gastric surgery for severe obesity." Publication No. 96-4006, 1996.

National Institutes of Health. "Very low-calorie diets." Publication No. 95-3894, 1995.

National Institutes of Health, National Hear, Lung and Blood Institute. "Clinical guidelines on the identification, evaluation and treatment of overweight and obesity in adults." *The Evidence Report*, 1998.

National Institutes of Health: Weight-control Information Network. www.niddk.nig.gov/health/nutrit/win.htm

Reaven, G. M. "Do high carbohydrate diets prevent the development or attenuate the manifestations (or both) of syndrome X? a viewpoint stronly against." *Current Opinions in Lipidology* 8 no. 1 (1997): 23.

Reaven, G. M. "Syndrome X." *Clinical Diabetes* 12 (1994): 32.

Rolls, B. J. and Hill, J. O. *Carbohydrates and Weight Management.* International Life Sciences Institute. Washington D.C.: ILSI Press, 1998.

Schlundt, D. G., et al. "Randomized evaluation of a low fat ad libitum carbo- hydrate diet for weight reduction." *International Journal of Obesity* 17 (1993): 623-39.

Sears, B. *Enter the Zone.* New York: Harper Collins, 1995.

Shah, M. et al. "Comparison of a low-fat, ad libitum complex-carbohydrate diet with a low-energy diet in moderately obese women." *American Journal of Clinical Nutrition* 59 (1994): 980-84.

Steward, H. L., C. B. Morrison, S. S. Andrew, et al. *Sugar Busters.* Ballantine Books, 1998.

Tiwary, C. M., J. A. Ward, B. A. Jackson. "Effect of pectin on satiety in healthy US Army adults." *Journal of the American College of Nutrition* 16 no. 5 (1997): 423-38.

Toth, M. J. and Poehlman, E. T. "Sympathetic nervous system activity and resting metabolic rate in vegetarians." *Metabolism* 43 no. 5 (1994): 621-25.

World Health Organization. "Obesity: Preventing and Managing the Global Epidemic: Report of a WHO Consultation of Obesity." Geneva, Switzerland: World Health Organization; 1997.

World Health Organization. *The World Health Report 1998.* www.who.int/whr/1998/whr-en.htm

Chapter 5

American Diabetes Association. "Evidence-based nutrition principles and rec- ommendations for the treatment and prevention of diabetes and related complications." *Diabetes Care* 25 (2002): 148-198.

American Dietetic Association and Dietitians of Canada. *Manual of Clinical Dietetics,* 6th ed. Chicago: American Dietetic Association, 2000.

Davis, B. and V. Melina. *Becoming Vegan.* Summertown TN: Book Publishing Co., 2000.

Food and Nutrition Board Institute of Medicine. *Dietary Reference Intakes.* National Academy Press. Washington DC. Available online at: http://www.nap.edu/index.html

Gorden, D. *Vegetarian Nutrition Guide.* Ypsilanti, MI: Dennis Gorden, 1997.

Pennington, J. A. *Bowes and Church's Food Values of Portions Commonly Used.* 16th ed. Philadelphia: J. B. Lippincott Co, 1994.

USDA Nutrient Database for Standard Reference at:
www.nal.usda.gov/fnic/cgi-bin/nut_search.pl

Chapter 6

American Diabetes Association. "Evidence-based nutrition principles and recommendations for the treatment and prevention of diabetes and related complications." *Diabetes Care* 25 (2002): 148-198.

American Dietetic Association. "Use of nutritive and non-nutritive sweeteners: Position of the American Dietetic Association." *Journal of the American Dietetic Association* 98 (1998): 580-87.

American Dietetic Association and Dietitians of Canada. *Manual of Clinical Dietetics*, 6th ed. Chicago: American Dietetic Association, 2000.

Bradstock, M., M. Serdula, M., J. Marks, et al. "Evaluation of reactions to food additives: The aspartame experience." *American Journal of Clinical Nutrition* 43 (1986): 464-69.

Center for Science in the Public Interest Website: http://www.cspinet.org/

Cicinelli-Timm, D. "What are polyols and how do they work into diabetes meal plans?" *Diabetes Care and Education* 21 no. 5 (2000): 10-16.

Committee on the Evaluation of Cyclamate and Carcinogenicity. *Evaluation of Cyclamate for Carcinogenicity*. Washington, DC: National Academy of Science, National Resource Council, 1985.

Council on Scientific Affairs, American Medical Association. "Saccharin: Review of safety issues." *Journal of the American Medical Association* 254 (1985): 2622-24.

Council on Scientific Affairs, American Medical Association. "Aspartame: Review of safety issues." *Journal of the American Medical Association* 254 (1985): 400-02.

FDA Statement on Aspartame. Rockville, MD: Food and Drug Administration. FDA Talk Paper. November 18, 1996.

Food and Drug Administration. "Health claims: Dietary sugar alcohols and dental caries." *Federal Register* 61 (August 23, 1996): 43433-445.

Garriga, M., C. Berkebile, D. Metcalfe. "A combined single-blind, double-blind, placebo-controlled study to determine the reproducibility of hypersensitivity reactions to aspartame." *Journal of Allergy and Clinical Immunology* 87 (1991): 821-27.

Glinsmann, W. and Park. Y. "Perspective on the 1986 Food and Drug Administration assessment of the safety of carbohydrate sweeteners: Uniform definitions and recommendations for future assessments." *American Journal of Clinical Nutrition* 62 (1995): 161S-169S.

Health Hazard Evaluation. "Summary of Adverse Reactions Attributed to Aspartame." Washington, DC: US Dept of Health and Human Services, 1995.

Joint FAO/WHO Expert Committee on Food Additives. "Toxicological Evaluation of Certain Food Additives." WHO Food Additives Series 42: 119-43, Geneva, 1999.

Kojima, S. and Ichibagase, H. "Cyclohexylamine, a metabolite of sodium cyclamate." *Chemical Pharmacology Bulletin* 14 (1966): 971-74.

London, R. "Saccharin and aspartame. Are they safe to consume during pregnancy?" *Journal of Reproductive Medicine* 33 no. 1 (1988): 17-21.

Mackey, S. and Berlin, C. J. "Effect of dietary aspartame on plasma concentrations of phenylalanine and tyrosine in normal and homozygous phenylketonuric patients." *Clinical Pediatrics* 31 (1992): 394-99.

Maher, T., R. Wurtman. "Possible neurological effects of aspartame, a widely used food additive." *Environmental Health Perspectives* 75 (1987): 53-57.

Malerbi, D., E. Paiva, E., A. Duarte, et al. "Metabolic effects of dietary sucrose and fructose in type II diabetic subjects." *Diabetes Care* 19 (1996): 1249-56.

Morgan, R. and Wong, O. "A review of epidemiological studies on artificial sweeteners and bladder cancer." *Food Chemisty Toxicology* 23 (1985): 529-33.

Pitkin, R. M., W/ Reynolds, L. J. Filer, et al. "Placental transmission and fetal distribution of saccharin." *American Journal of Obstetrics and Gynecology* 111 (1971): 280-86.

Price, J., B. Blava, B. Oser, et al. "Bladder tumors in rats fed cyclohexylamine or high doses of a mixture of cyclamate and saccharin." *Science* 167 (1970): 1131-32.

Ranney, R., J. Oppermann, E. Muldoon, et al. "Comparative metabolism of aspartame in experimental animals and humans." *Journal of Toxicology and Environmental Health* 2 (1976): 441-51.

Risch, H. "Dietary factors and the incidence of cancer of the urinary bladder." *American Journal of Epidemiology* 127 (1988): 1179-91.

Rowan, A., B. Shaywitz, L. Tuchman, et al. "Aspartame and seizure susceptibility: results of a clinical study in reportedly sensitive individuals." *Epilepsia* 36 (1995): 270-75.

Scientific Committee on Food. European Commission, Consumer Policy and Consumer Health Protection. "Opinion on stevioside as a sweetener." 1999.

Stegink, L. and Filer, L. J. "Effects of aspartame ingestion on plasma aspartate, phenylalanine, and methanol concentrations in normal adults." In *The Clinical Evaluation of a Food Additive.* edited by C. Tschanz, et al. New York: CRC Press, 1996.

Wasuntarawat, C., P. Temcharoen, C. Toskulkao, et al. "Developmental toxicity of steviol, a metabolite of stevioside, in the hamster." *Drug Chemistry and Toxicology* 21 no. 2 (May 1998): 207-22.

Weil, Dr. Andrew. Website: http://www.drweil.com/

Wolever, T. and Brand, J. "Sugars and blood glucose control." *American Journal of Clinical Nutrition* 62 (1995): 212S-227S.

Chapter 7

American Diabetes Association. "Evidence-based nutrition principles and recommendations for the treatment and prevention of diabetes and related complications." *Diabetes Care* 25 (2002): 148-198.

American Dietetic Association and Dietitians of Canada. *Manual of Clinical Dietetics*, 6th ed. Chicago: American Dietetic Association, 2000.

Johnson, R. K. and Frary, C. "Choose beverages and foods to moderate your intake of sugars: the 2000 dietary guidelines for Americans—what's all the fuss about?" *Journal of Nutrition* 131 no. 10 (October 2001): 2766S-71S.

Pennington, J. A. *Bowes and Church's Food Values of Portions Commonly Used*. 16th ed. Philadelphia: J. B. Lippincott Co, 1994.

USDA Nutrient Database for Standard Reference at: http://www.nal.usda.gov/fnic/cgi-bin/nut_search.pl

Warshaw, H. "Healthy restaurant eating: Is it possible?" The American Diabetes Association Website: http://www.diabetes.org/main/health/nutrition/restauranteating.jsp

Index

Recipe titles and table references are shown in italics.